Nursing Quality Indicators Beyond Acute Care

Literature Review

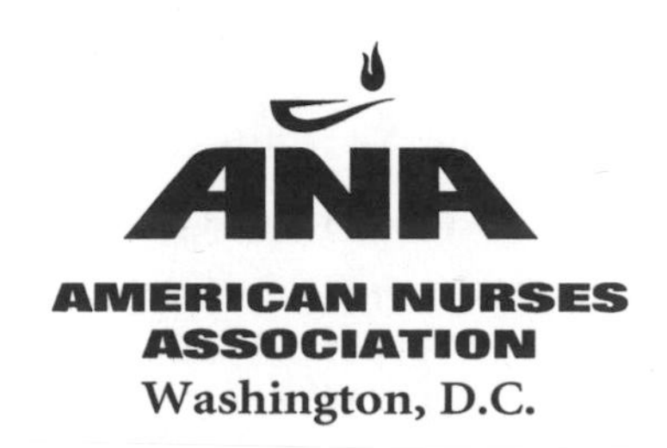

AMERICAN NURSES ASSOCIATION
Washington, D.C.

Library of Congress Cataloging-in-Publication Data

Nursing quality indicators beyond acute care: literature review.
p. ; cm.
Includes bibliographical references.
ISBN 1-55810-149-7
1. Nursing–Standards–Miscellanea. 2. Nursing–Quality control–Miscellanea.
3. Quality assurance–Miscellanea. I. American Nurses Association.
[DNLM: 1. Nursing Care–standards. 2. Quality Indicators, Health Care.
WY 100 N97857 2000]
RT85.5 .N8664 2000
610.73'02'18—dc21

00-033186

Published by
American Nurses Publishing
600 Maryland Avenue, SW
Suite 100 West
Washington, DC 20024-2571

ISBN 1-55810-149-7

LR20 2M 12/00

Acknowledgments

Advisory Committee for Community-based Nonacute Care Indicators

Linda M. Sawyer, PhD, RN, CS
QISMC Manager, CMRI

Bobbie Berkowitz, PhD, RN, FAAN
Director, RWJF Turning Point NPO
Professor and Chair, Department of Psychosocial and Community Health
School of Nursing, University of Washington

Judith E. Haber, PhD, APRN, CS, FAAN
Visiting Professor, Director of Master's and Post-Master's Certificate Programs
Division of Nursing, New York University

June H. Larrabee, PhD, RN
Associate Professor, West Virginia University School of Nursing
Clinical Investigator, West Virginia Hospitals

Barbara L. Marino, PhD, RN
Trustee, American Nurses Foundation

Karen S. Martin, RN, MSN, FAAN
Health Care Consultant

Katherine P. Mason, MPH, RN, EdD
Council on Community, Primary, and Long Term Care Nursing
Director of Performance Improvement, Florida Department of Health

Margaret F. Mastal, PhD, MSN, RN
Chief Operating Officer
Health Services for Children with Special Needs, Inc.

Michael W. Nilsson, RN
Pasco County (Florida) Health Department

Sue Ellen Walbridge
Office of Science, U. S. Department of Energy

Mary K. Walker, PhD, RN, FAAN
Dean, School of Nursing, University of Seattle

Committee Technical Advisors

Barbara Holtzclaw, PhD, RN, FAAN
School of Nursing, University of Texas Health Science Center

Norma M. Lang, PhD, RN, FRCN, FAAN
Dean, School of Nursing, University of Pennsylvania

Pamela Mitchell, PhD, CNRN, FAAN
Adjunct Professor, Department of Health Services
School of Nursing, University of Washington

Vector Research Inc.

Deborah Coley

Mary Fisher

Katherine Jones

Michelle Banfield

American Nursing Association

Patricia Rowell, PhD, RN
Senior Policy Fellow, Nursing Practice

Yvonne Humes, BBA
Senior Administrative Assistant

Contents

Background

The current corporatization of health care has resulted in increased emphasis on cost-cutting measures that have had an adverse impact on Registered Nurses (RNs) providing patient/client care services. The American Nurses Association (ANA) has initiated work in a number of areas to explore the relationship between RN staffing and safety and quality of client care. These efforts have included far-reaching public relations efforts such as the "Every Patient Deserves a Nurse" campaign, political activities, public testimony such as the Joint Commission for Accreditation of Healthcare Organizations (JCAHO) restraint hearings, and other work with public officials and policy makers.

A critical and pioneering component of this work has been research to examine relationships between RN staffing, processes of care and patient outcomes in acute care. In 1994 when ANA launched Nursing's Safety and Quality Initiative (the Initiative), limited research exploring the relationship between staffing and patient/client outcomes was available. The ANA Board of Directors determined that ANA must lead the nursing community in the design and implementation of ongoing, comprehensive, broad-based research efforts to establish and quantify the impact of RN staffing on processes of care and patient/client outcomes; thus, Nursing's Safety and Quality Initiative.

In undertaking the research component of the Initiative, the initial step was to decide that the indicators would measure the input of nursing practice to patient/client outcomes rather than the individual nurse's contributions. Thus, ANA's indicators are nursing-sensitive rather than nurse-sensitive indicators. Initially, the identification of nursing-sensitive indicators focused upon the acute care setting; the need for indicators to measure nursing's input to patient/client care across the continuum, however, was always clear. In 1994, an Advisory Committee to develop acute care indicators was appointed. That Advisory Committee completed identification of the acute care indicators in 1995 and published them in *Nursing's Acute Care Report Card* (ANA 1995). Following publication, a three-year process of pilot testing the indicators was undertaken. In 2000, there are approximately 120 hospitals participating in the collection of data. In addition, the National Database of Nursing Quality Indicators (NDNQI), the repository for the nursing-sensitive data collected in this project, was established and serves as the analyzer of the data. At this point in time, data collection for acute care facilities is ongoing.

In 1997, the Advisory Committee for Community-based Nonacute Care Indicators to identify indicators sensitive to the impact of nursing practice in community-based nonacute settings was appointed by the ANA Congress of Nursing Practice. In late 1999, the Advisory Committee identified and the Congress of Nursing Practice and Economics approved ten nursing-sensitive indicators for community-based nonacute settings. Those indicators are:

- **Pain management (symptom severity)**—The treatment and prevention of pain and discomfort. Effectiveness is related to the level of functioning and the activities of daily living and includes measures of frequency, intensity, and duration of pain symptoms.
- **Consistency of communication (strength of therapeutic alliance)**—Consistent RN/APRN provider identified in the data/record.
- **Staff mix (utilization of services)**—Total number of direct care hours or total number of encounters provided by RN or advanced practice registered nurse (APRN) staff who have client care responsibilities (per episode/encounter/case as appropriate to the setting) determined as follows:
    - *Primary measure (RNs, LPNs, and UAPs caring for clients)* —The percent of registered nursing care hours as a total of all nursing care hours.
    - *Secondary measure*—The percent of APRNs.
    - *Client satisfaction*—The degree to which the care received met client expectations regarding nursing care, pain management, patient education, and overall care.
- **Prevention of tobacco use (risk reduction)**—Number of clients attending educational sessions per year provided and/or coordinated by RNs about the risks of tobacco use (includes coordination of educational sessions/programs either with individuals or groups).
- **Cardiovascular prevention (risk reduction)**—Number of clients attending educational sessions per year provided and/or coordinated by RNs about risks of cardiovascular disease.
- **Care giver activity (protective factors)**—Existence or frequency of primary care giver involvement.
- **Identification of primary care giver (protective factors).**
- **ADL/IADL (level of function)** — The degree to which the normal physical or entire action of a system occurs (physical or psychological).
- **Psychosocial interaction (level of function)** —The degree to which the normal action of a system occurs.

Methodology

The methods used to identify the community-based nonacute indicators are consistent with the recommended methodology for development of evidence-based documents of the Agency for Healthcare Research and Quality (formerly the Agency for Health Care Policy and Research). The same methods were used for identification of ANA's acute care indicators.

A thorough review of the literature was conducted using the following criteria:

- Is the research scientifically sound? If not, what are the research's limitations?
- Is the research valid and reliable?
- Is the indicator sensitive to nursing intervention?
- Are the data retrievable?
- Is the operational definition included? If so, what is the definition?

A complete and proper citation for each study was required. If the above five criteria were not met, the study was not included in the review.

Following the Advisory Committee's identification of potential indicators, expert clinicians reviewed the indicators and recommended those they thought would have the greatest utility and were collectable. Following that input, the Advisory Committee made its decisions.

Theoretical Overview

Avedis Donabedian's model of structure, process and outcome guided the work of the ANA Advisory Committee for Acute Care Indicators as they identified indicators of quality of nursing care for acutely ill patients. In his model, Donabedian proposes that client outcomes are related to the care processes and to the structures of care. However, structures and processes may affect outcomes directly, indirectly, and/or cumulatively. It is, therefore, important to take structures, processes, and outcomes into consideration when trying to understand quality of patient care.

The Advisory Committee for Community-based Nonacute Care Indicators strove to be consistent with the work of the previous committee. Seeking indicators that reflect the quality of nursing care, the Advisory Committee acknowledged that the set of indicators should include measures of structure (such as skill mix), nursing process and client outcomes (that is, outcomes that have a strong relationship to nursing care). During the Advisory Committee's first meeting, a presentation of Evan's and Stoddard's model[1] that places the health of an individual or a community in the context of many intrinsic and community influences broadened the members' conceptualization of the work they were about to undertake. With this model, health care is only one of many factors influencing health and illness. Evan's and Stoddard's thinking reinforced the Advisory Committee's intent to select client outcomes carefully: only outcomes that have clear links to nursing care should be selected as indicators of nursing-sensitive care.

---

[1]Institute of Medicine. 1997. *Improving Health in the Community.* Washington, DC: National Academy Press, pp. 45–56.

The literature search was, therefore, designed to find empirical evidence of links between nursing care in the community and client outcomes. In reviewing the literature, eight areas of interest for which indicators thought to be sensitive to nursing care input were identified:

1. Change in symptom severity
2. Level of functioning
3. Strength of the therapeutic alliance
4. Utilization of services
5. Client/patient satisfaction
6. Risk reduction (environmental, behavioral)
7. Increase in protective factors (that is, behaviors where the individual or family seek information and a support system and, ultimately, act on the knowledge derived from this involvement)
8. Satisfaction with quality of life

The following literature review is that which the Advisory Committee generated and used in its work to identify nursing-sensitive indicators for community-based nonacute care clients.

Introduction

Vector Research Incorporated (VRI), was contracted by the American Nurses Association (ANA) to prepare a literature review and annotated bibliography of the research-based literature on indicators sensitive to the quality or availability of nursing care in eight areas. These areas were identified by an ANA advisory committee as being synonymous with quality care and sensitive to variations in the quality or availability of nursing care in settings other than acute care. The following are the eight areas of interest:

- Changes in symptom severity
- Level of functioning
- Strength of the therapeutic alliance
- Utilization of services
- Patient/client satisfaction
- Risk reduction (environmental/behavioral)
- Increase in protective factors
- Satisfaction with quality of life

Following the literature review, VRI analyzed the scientific merit of the identified indicators.

The review of the research-based literature produced a myriad of studies on health outcomes and quality of care as well as a variety of scales to measure these concepts. This analysis was into two parts. During the first part of the analysis, articles and academic publications were reviewed that contained references to quality care, quality indicators, nursing care, and patient outcomes. By reviewing these texts, the most commonly cited indicators were identified an empirical or theoretical link to the eight areas identified by ANA and the availability or quality of nursing care. Appendix A contains a checklist of the identified indicators and the criteria used to evaluate their scientific merit.

The second phase of the literature review focused on locating articles that could be used to analyze the scientific merit of the indicators. For the annotated bibliography, VRI abstracted articles by obtaining the following information:

- Purpose of the study
- Description of the sample
- Methods and data analysis
- Time frame of the study
- Findings (including the statistical significance, if noted)
- Relationship between the indicator and nursing care
- Relevance of the findings to settings other than acute care
- Any study limitations

Because some of the indicators appear under more than one category, there was some overlap in the indicators identified for each of the areas, and some of the articles will be referenced in multiple places in the subsequent annotated bibliography. In the second phase of the literature review, focusing on identifying indicators sensitive to the quality or availability of nursing care for the eight areas identified by ANA significantly reduced the available literature, since very little of it focused directly on nursing care. For this reason, a broad base of literature was used to evaluate the relationship of the indicators to the eight identified areas and the scientific merit of the indicators. Nursing-specific literature was relied on to relate the indicators to the quality or availability of nursing care. Sensitivity to nursing interventions or nursing practice was used as a proxy for sensitivity to the quality or availability of nursing care. Appendix B contains the annotated bibliography.

The following analysis (in Chapters 1–8) focuses on identifying and analyzing the research-based literature, assessing the scientific merit of the indicators, evaluating their relationship to the eight areas of interest, and demonstrating their sensitivity to the availability or quality of nursing care. The analysis was broken into eight parts to coincide with the eight areas of interest to ANA. Only the indicators displaying some evidence to support their scientific merit were included in the analysis beyond a passing reference. The indicators are rank ordered, beginning with the indicator with the strongest support in the research-based literature. The checklist in Appendix A was used to record two factors: (1) achievement of the criterion used to evaluate the scientific merit of the indicators and (2) moderately supported linkages to the criteria that were made in the studies.

There was a large amount of variability in the degree to which the research-based literature could demonstrate the scientific merit of the original potential indicators. Several of the identified indicators do not appear in the detailed analysis because there was insufficient scientific evidence to support their inclusion. Other indicators showed some evidence of scientific merit but were lacking in studies linking them to the availability or quality of nursing care or settings other than acute care. Indicators with strong scientific merit but a weak link to nursing in settings other than acute care included the following: symptom management/relief (fluid and electrolyte status), symptom management/

relief (skin integrity), symptom management/relief (continence), symptom management/relief (cognition/sensory deficits/orientation), performance of activities of daily living/instrumental activities of daily living (ADLs/IADLs), satisfaction with staff mix, and self-efficacy.

The following lists include the indicators of moderately strong scientific merit that possess a demonstrated linkage to the quality or availability of nursing care and a linkage to settings other than acute care, categorized according to Donabedian's framework of structure, process, and outcomes. Due to the fine lines between these three categories, several indicators appear in somewhat modified forms under more than one category.

Patient-Focused Outcome Indicators

- Change in the severity of symptoms of altered respiratory status
- Change in the severity of symptoms of altered nutritional/oral status
- Frequency/intensity/duration of symptoms (percent of time spent in improved/worsened state)
- Level of physical functioning (exercise tolerance, ambulation, mobility, and transferring)
- Level of psychological/neurological/cognitive functioning
- Level of psychosocial functioning (emotional, behavioral, social interaction)
- Satisfaction with access to timeliness of care
- Patient satisfaction with communication
- Patient participation in healthcare management (medications and treatments)
- Number of emergency room visits
- Satisfaction with quality of nursing care rendered
- Patient adherence to exercise regimen
- Weight control/loss–appropriate dietary intake
- Rate of patient injury/falls

Structure of Care Indicators: Patient-centered Care

- Coordination of care processes/continuity of care
- Consistency, timeliness, and style of communication
- Patient/family involvement in care planning/decision-making
- Appropriateness of emergency room visits
- Existence/frequency of involvement of a primary caregiver

Process of Care Indicators

- Pain management
- Management/relief of symptoms of altered respiratory status
- Management/relief of symptoms of altered nutritional/oral status
- Coordination of care processes/continuity of care
- Number/appropriateness of clinic visits
- Number of home visits

- Consistency, timeliness, and style of communication
- Prevention of injury/falls

The remainder of this document presents the specifics of the analysis of the scientific merit of these indicators. More detail about each indicator can be found by reviewing the annotated bibliographies for the referenced articles in Appendix B. Appendix A presents a quick overview of the findings. Appendix C contains references used to identify nursing quality indicators. Appendix D lists other literature that was reviewed but not included in the annotated bibliography.

Changes in Symptom Severity 1

For purposes of this research, change in symptom severity was defined as the degree to which a patient's experience of the subjective evidence of their disease or illness varies. The indicators are focused on frequency, intensity, and duration of symptoms such as pain, edema/fluid retention, nausea/ vomiting, shortness of breath, and pruritis. All of the identified potential quality indicators for changes in symptom severity had supporting literature; therefore, none were excluded from this analysis.

Symptom Management/Relief (Pain Management/Physical Comfort–Degree of Pain)

Six studies supported the use of symptom management/relief of pain indicators for measuring change in symptom severity. Coenen et al. (1995), McCloskey and Bulechek (1995), Rosenthal et al. (1992), Stucki et al. (1996), and Vines et al. (1996) demonstrated the validity of pain measurement tools for measuring changes in symptom severity. The Rosenthal et al., Vines et al., and Stucki et al. studies further demonstrated that the tools were reliable, sensitive, and responsive. Peruselli et al. (1997) also demonstrated sensitivity and responsiveness of pain measurement tools for patients in a home palliative care service. The link between nursing care and tools to measure pain severity was demonstrated in the Coenen et al. (1995), Peruselli et al., Rosenthal et al., and McCloskey and Bulechek articles in that nursing staff conducted the pain-severity assessment and were generally the ones responsible for pain management. The link between the pain assessment tools and use in the nonacute care settings was supported by articles (Peruselli et al. 1997); the other studies were conducted in acute care settings. These studies assessed patients with cancer in community settings, patients admitted to an academic center, and patients undergoing surgery at an academic center, demonstrating that pain management indicators may be generalizable across settings. The limitations of these studies were that some did not demonstrate a clear link to nursing, three were conducted in acute care settings, one was based on the opinions of nurses and not a clinical trial, and one was based on a small sample size.

Symptom Management/Relief (Fluid and Electrolyte Status)

Five studies supported the change in fluid and electrolyte status as a measure for symptom severity. All five studies (Coenen et al. 1995; McCloskey and Bulechek 1995; Rantz et al. 1997), Rosenthal et al. 1992; Visalli 1997) validated the use of fluid status changes as an indicator for symptom severity, and the interventions were linked to nursing care. The Rantz study demonstrated a link between this indicator and nursing care in a long-term care setting. The Rosenthal et al. study further demonstrated the reliability of this indicator but did so in the acute care setting. The Coenen et al., Rantz, and Rosenthal et al. studies demonstrated the sensitivity and responsiveness of this indicator in long-term and acute care settings. The generalizability of the results is demonstrated by the variety of clinical conditions represented by the sample groups, but their applicability to nonacute care settings was not specifically addressed. The Visalli study was limited by the lack of detailed description of the design, subjects, methodology, and data analysis used to conduct the study.

Symptom Management/Relief (Skin Integrity)

Three studies supported the use of symptom management/relief of altered skin integrity as an indicator for measuring change in symptom severity. All three studies (McCloskey and Bulechek; 1995; Rantz et al. 1997; Rosenthal et al. 1992) validated the use of skin integrity indicators for measuring changes in symptom severity. As with other indicators for change in symptom severity, the Rosenthal et al. study further demonstrated the reliability in acute care settings, and the Rosenthal et al. and Rantz studies demonstrated the sensitivity and responsiveness of the indicator in acute and long-term care settings, respectively. Due to the variety of clinical conditions represented by the sample groups, the results from the studies are generalizable to a variety of clinical conditions. All three studies linked the indicator to the quality or availability of nursing care. Other limitations of the studies for this indicator were that one was conducted in an acute care setting, and the other was not a clinical trial study but a survey of professional nurses' opinions.

Symptom Management/Relief (Respiratory Status)

Three articles from the literature review supported the use of symptom management/relief for respiratory status as an indicator for measuring change in symptom severity (McCloskey and Bulechek 1995; Rosenthal et al. 1992; Peruselli et al. 1997). McCloskey and Bulechek (1995) and Rosenthal et al. demonstrated the validity of respiratory status as an indicator for symptom severity. Rosenthal et al. further demonstrated the reliability, sensitivity, and responsiveness of the indicator, with Peruselli et al. adding further support of sensitivity and responsiveness. A link to nursing was apparent from all three studies, and the study by Peruselli et al. supported a link to practice in nonacute care settings. Furthermore, the variety of clinical conditions represented in the studies supported the generalizability of this indicator.

Symptom Management/Relief (Nutritional/Oral Status, Including Nausea/Vomiting)

Six studies determined that nutrition, oral status, nausea, and vomiting were measures of change in symptom severity. Four studies (Graham et al. 1993; McCloskey and Bulechek 1995; Rantz et al. 1997; and Rosenthal et al. 1992) validated the use of these indicators for measuring changes in symptom severity. The Rosenthal et al. study further demonstrated reliability, sensitivity, and responsiveness of these indicators. Perucelli (1997) and Rantz (1997) also demonstrated sensitivity and responsiveness; Smith (1994) demonstrated sensitivity only. All of the studies demonstrated a link to nursing care, but only the Perucelli and Rantz studies clearly linked the nursing interventions to nonacute care. The generalizability of the results is demonstrated by the variety of clinical conditions represented by the studies. The Graham study was limited by the fact that statistical tests of significance were not conducted.

Frequency/Duration/Intensity of Symptoms (Percentage of Time Spent in Improved/Worsened State)

Three studies related to the frequency, intensity, or duration of symptoms (Perucelli et al. 1997; Rosenthal et al. 1992; Stucki et al. 1996). Only the study by Rosenthal et al. demonstrated the validity and reliability of using indicators of frequency, duration, or intensity of symptoms to measure change in symptom severity. All three studies demonstrated the sensitivity of these indicators to clinically significant change over time. Responsiveness and link to nursing care were demonstrated in the Perucelli and Rosenthal et al. studies. As with other indicators in the area of change in symptom severity, the generalizability of the results is demonstrated by the variety of clinical conditions represented in the subjects. The Perucelli study, however, was the only study that was linked to nursing in the nonacute care setting. The limitations of these studies have been mentioned in previous sections.

Symptom Management/Relief (Continence)

Two studies related to continence and the change in symptom severity. McCloskey and Bulechek. (1995) and Rosenthal et al. (1992) both validated the continence measures as indicators for change in symptom severity. The Rosenthal et al. study further demonstrated the reliability, sensitivity, and responsiveness of continence measures. Generalizability of this indicator was demonstrated by the variety of conditions represented in the group of subjects. Links to nursing care were demonstrated in both studies; however, links to settings other than acute care were not clearly established.

Symptom Management/Relief (Cognition/Sensory Deficits/Orientation)

The literature contained five studies related to the change in cognitive/sensory perception (Baradell [1995; Campbell 1992; McCloskey and Bulechek 1995; Rosenthal et al. 1992; Brietbart 1997). Indicators that measure changes in cognitive status were validated in all five studies. Reliability was demonstrated in the Rosenthal et al. and Brietbart studies, and sensitivity and responsiveness were shown in the Rantz and Rosenthal et al. studies. The generalizability of the results is demonstrated by the variety of clinical conditions represented by the sample groups. The Baradell, Campbell, Rosenthal et al., and McCloskey and Bulechek studies also showed the link to nursing care, and the Baradell and Campbell studies showed a link to nonacute care nursing.

There are numerous studies supporting the strength of the scientific merit of all of the identified indicators in this area. It can be assumed that symptom severity and the treatment of symptoms are similar in acute and nonacute care settings. There is limited research on changes in symptom severity in settings other than acute care. Furthermore, the many valid and reliable methods and tools that exist for measuring symptom severity are generally not nursing-specific; therefore, there may be confounding factors that make it difficult to assess the precise impact of the quality or availability of nursing care on the changes in symptom severity.

Level of Functioning 2

For the purposes of this research, level of functioning was defined as the degree to which the normal or proper action of a limb, organ, or entire system occurs, or any deviation from that norm. The quality indicators in this area focus on physical, psychosocial, role, and cognitive functioning, with an emphasis on those indicators most sensitive to nursing care. Participation in healthcare management (medication and treatment), role performance, and maintenance/improvement in functioning were identified as potential nursing quality indicators; however, the literature review produced insufficient evidence to support the use of these indicators as measures of patient level of functioning. Therefore, no further analyses were conducted on these indicators.

Activities of Daily Living/Instrumental Activities of Daily Living (ADLs/IADLs)

A considerable amount of literature supporting the use of this indicator in non-acute nursing care quality assessment practices was found. The Whittle and Goldenberg study (1996) determined that IADLs were a valid measure of both physical and social functioning for older patients being cared for in their homes with a variety of chronic health conditions. Ottenbacher et al. (1994) showed that IADLs were reliable measures for community-based elderly by reporting the strong inter-rater reliability. Furthermore, Peruselli et al. (1997) demonstrated the sensitivity and responsiveness of ADLs for cancer patients receiving care either in an outpatient clinic or in their home. These studies also demonstrated that ADLs/IADLs can be linked to nursing care in nonacute care settings and are generalizable to a large group of older adults in community-based settings being treated for a variety of health conditions. Some of the limits of the research include the fact that some studies used small sample sizes and some studies were not nursing-specific. ADLs/IADLs are accepted as a relatively standard and validated method of measuring patient level of functioning. The questions contained in the ADL/IADL related directly to everyday activities. There are valid tools available, the measurement tools can be self-administered, and a person assessing these activities can ascertain an accurate level of functioning from observation or questioning of the patient and/or family members.

Physical Functioning (Exercise Tolerance, Ambulation, Mobility, and Transferring)

Four studies assessed physical functioning as an indicator for level of functioning. Gortner and Jenkins (1990), McCloskey and Bulechek (1995), Stucki et al. (1996), and Whittle and Goldenberg. (1996) each validated physical functioning as an indicator for patient level of functioning. Stucki et al. further demonstrated the reliability, sensitivity, and responsiveness of physical functioning indicators on patients undergoing surgery in a hospital setting. The study by Gortner and Jenkins further demonstrated reliability and responsiveness of the indicator for cardiac surgery patients. McCloskey and Bulechek surveyed a group of nurses on the usefulness of Nursing Interventions Classifications (NICs) taxonomy structure of which physical functioning is a part, demonstrating a link of physical functioning indicators to nursing care. Making a link to nonacute care practice setting and demonstrating generalizability, Whittle studied noninstitutionalized elderly with a variety of clinical conditions who were being cared for in family practice clinics. Gortner and Jenkins also showed links between the indicator and nursing care and between the indicator and care delivered in nonacute settings. Many valid and reliable tools/methods for measuring physical functioning and changes in physical functioning are available.

Psychological/Neurological/Cognitive Functioning

Five studies related psychological indicators to overall patient level of functioning (Abraham and Reel et al. 1992; Baradell 1995; Brietbart et al. 1997; McCloskey and Bulechek 1995; Peruselli et al. 1997). All five studies validated the use of psychological/neurological/cognitive functioning as indicators of overall level of functioning and established a link between this indicator and the quality of availability of nursing care. Through the validation of the NIC structure, McCloskey and Bulechek determined that interventions to improve psychological functioning, including those related to cognitive therapy and psychological comfort promotion, were valid and effective for improving overall patient level of functioning. The Brietbart study (1997) went further, validating not only the use of cognitive indicators for measuring psychological functioning but their reliability as well. The Abraham and Reel study further demonstrated the sensitivity, reliability, and responsiveness of this indicator. Peruselli et al. (1997) demonstrated that the severity of psychological measures changed over time and that psychological factors were responsive to nursing interventions. Furthermore, Abraham and Reel, Baradell, Peruselli et al., and McCloskey and Bulechek established the link between psychological functioning and nursing care in nonacute care settings. The generalizability of these findings was demonstrated by the variety of clinical conditions represented by the study subjects. There are several valid and reliable methods and tools for assessing psychological, neurological, and cognitive functioning.

Psychosocial Functioning

Four studies supported the psychosocial measures as indicators for overall patient level of functioning. All four studies (Baradell 1995; Smits 1992; Stucki et al. 1996; Whittle 1996) validated the use of psychosocial indicators for measuring patient level of functioning. Stucki et al. further demonstrated the reliability, sensitivity, and responsiveness of psychosocial indicators. Baradell and Smits demonstrated a link between psychosocial indicators and nursing care in non-acute care settings and concluded that psychosocial indicators were generalizable. The use of psychosocial indicators of functioning in nonacute care settings was also conducted in the Whittle study. The weaknesses of the studies identified for this indicator were that two of them (Smits; Stucki et al.) did not look at the impact of nursing interventions on psychosocial functioning, and only one study (Stucki et al.) verified reliability, sensitivity, and responsiveness of the measure. Many methods and tools are available that have demonstrated validity and reliability with respect to psychosocial functioning.

All of the indicators analyzed had fairly strong scientific merit; however, more research may be needed to establish a link between physical functioning and the quality or availability of nursing care. There are many proven tools and methods for measuring these indicators; however, it may be difficult to measure the impact of the availability or quality of nursing care on the measures.

Strength of the Therapeutic Alliance

3

For purpose of this research, *strength of the therapeutic alliance* was defined as the degree to which a positive relationship exists between the patient, family, or other caregivers, and clinicians, demonstrating comprehensive, patient-centered, coordinated care that is well communicated, acceptable, and timely. Trust between patient and providers, comprehensive care, integration of care, and accuracy of information were all identified as potential nursing-sensitive quality indicators; however, our literature review produced no evidence to support their use as measures of the strength of the therapeutic alliance. Therefore, no further analyses were conducted on these indicators.

Coordination of Care Processes/Continuity of Care

Three studies supported the use of coordination of care as an indicator for the strength of therapeutic alliance (Brooten et al. 1986; Burns et al.1996; Naylor et al. 1994). One of the studies (Burns et al.) supported the validity and reliability of coordination of care indicators for the strength of therapeutic alliance. All three demonstrated the responsiveness of the indicator, but none of the studies demonstrated sensitivity. Burns et al. showed that the indicator is generalizable in that their study was conducted on seniors with a variety of clinical conditions. Furthermore, the other study of mothers and infants (Brooten et al.) provides additional support for the generalizability of the indicator. All of the studies showed that the indicator has a direct link to nursing, but only the Burns et al. and Brooten et al. studies showed direct links to practice in non-acute care settings.

Communication: Consistency, Timeliness, and Style of Communication

Three studies supported the use of communication as an indicator of strength of the therapeutic alliance (Luborsky 1983; Barnard et al. 1988; Brown 1992).

Brown used communication by the nurse as an indicator for the strength of the therapeutic alliance. Luborsky (1983) looked at the communication style of patient and therapist to predict outcomes of psychotherapy. The Luborsky study supported the validity and reliability of communication as an indicator for the strength of therapeutic alliance. The Barnard et al. study demonstrated not only the validity but the sensitivity and responsiveness of this indicator. The Brown study further supported the generalizability of communication indicators. Links were made to nursing and nonacute care settings. Further studies are needed to determine the usefulness of this indicator as a measure for the strength of therapeutic alliance. The methods for measuring this indicator (such as taping conversations and deciphering patterns) were burdensome for the person conducting the evaluation.

Patient/Family Involvement in Care Planning and Decision-Making

Five studies suggested that patient family involvement was a reasonable indicator of the strength of the therapeutic alliance (Barnard et al. 1988; Brooten et al. 1986; Brown 1992; Szabo et al. 1997; Olds and Kitzman 1990). Four of the studies demonstrated the validity of the indicator as a measure for the strength of the therapeutic alliance, and the Barnard et al. study further demonstrated sensitivity and responsiveness; however, none of the studies demonstrated reliability. Olds and Kitzman and Brooten et al. demonstrated responsiveness of the indicator, and Brown demonstrated its generalizability. Links to nursing could be found in Barnard et al., Brown, Brooten et al., and Olds and Kitzman, as well as links to nonacute care settings. Brown focused specifically on testing patient/family involvement in care planning and decision-making. The other studies noted the success of interventions that incorporated a strong therapeutic alliance as a goal of the intervention. In the Brown study, the sample size was small and the method for measuring the indicator (taping conversations and deciphering patterns in taped conversations) was burdensome for the person conducting the investigation.

While some studies were located, the evidence found to support the scientific merit of the indicators in this area is weak. Further research is needed before using these indicators. Furthermore, the methods for measuring the indicators covered in the research were often time-consuming and very burdensome to the person measuring the indicator. Therefore, feasibility of the indicators may be questioned.

Utilization of Services 4

For purposes of this research, utilization of services was defined as the quantity or cost of health services used. The indicators focus on the impact on health service utilization (such as length of stay within the subacute care/ rehabilitation setting, outpatient visit rates, readmission rates, and emergency room visits) that is an outcome of the quality or availability of nursing care in nonacute care settings. Ambulatory-sensitive admission rate and number of visits per episode of care were identified as potential indicators of utilization of services; however, insufficient evidence was found to support the use of these indicators as a measure of use. Therefore, no further analyses were conducted on these indicators.

Number/Appropriateness of Clinic Visits

Five studies demonstrated how nursing interventions could impact clinic visits (Burns et al. 1996; Kitzman et al. 1997; Miller et al. 1996; Olds et al. 1995; Weinberger et al. 1996). Burns et al. demonstrated validity and reliability of clinic visits for measuring the impact of nursing interventions. The Kitzman et al. and Olds et al. studies further demonstrated the validity, sensitivity, and responsiveness of this indicator. All of the studies showed links between nursing care and use of clinic visits and links to healthcare delivery in nonacute care settings. Responsiveness and generalizability of this indicator were demonstrated in both the Burns et al. study and the Weinberger et al. study. Clinic visits are relatively easy to measure, particularly for patients who are enrolled in managed care organizations. Use of computerized databases to identify clinic visits is a common practice. IPA model HMOs, where clinicians submit claims to the HMO for reimbursement, would provide the most complete information about clinic visits for a given population. However, caution needs to be taken in determining the extent to which plan members may go outside the plan providers to obtain care, in which case there would not be a claim in the electronic databases for the visit.

Emergency Room Visits

Five studies supported the use of number/appropriateness of emergency room visits as an indicator for utilization (Burns et al. 1994; Brooten, Naylor et al. 1996; Kitzman et al. 1997; Miller et al. 1996; and Olds et al. 1995). The Burns et al. study demonstrated the validity and reliability of an emergency room indicator for utilization in response to nursing interventions. The Kitzman et al. and Olds et al. studies further demonstrated the validity, sensitivity, and responsiveness of this indicator. All of the studies demonstrated links to nursing care and to care that is delivered in nonacute care settings. Two of the other studies (Burns et al.; Miller et al.) showed that the indicator is responsive, although the trend was not found to be statistically significant in the Miller study. Generalizability of the indicator is supported by the Brooten et al. study in that they examined seven different patient groups, as well as by the Burns et al. study, which looked at a variety of clinical conditions in the elderly. Ease of measurement for this indicator is similar to clinic visits (see Number/Appropriateness of Clinic Visits section for a discussion on ease of measurement). However, specific codes and data for emergency or urgent care visits may vary by providers and institutions. Appropriate coding must be identified to use electronic data sources for emergency visit information. In addition, there are reliability issues with out-of-plan use of emergency rooms.

Readmissions

Five studies assessed how nursing interventions impacted readmission rates (Brooten et al. 1986; Naylor et al. 1994; Weinberger et al. 1996; Brooten, Naylor et al. 1996; Martens and Mellor 1997). All of the studies showed a link to nursing and a link to nonacute health service delivery settings. However, none of the studies tested the validity, reliability, or sensitivity of readmission rates as an indicator for utilization. All but the Brooten et al. (1996) study demonstrated the responsiveness of readmission rates to nursing interventions. Generalizability of the nursing interventions to impact readmission rates can be demonstrated by the variety of patient groups on which these interventions took place; that is, patients with congestive heart failure (CHF), patients who experienced unplanned caesarean delivery, very low birth weight infants, elderly people with medical cardiac diagnosis-related groups (DRGs), and people with surgical cardiac DRGs. As with clinic and emergency room visits, readmission rates may be difficult to measure, even with electronic database systems.

Number/Appropriateness of Home Health Visits

Four studies used home health visits as part of a nursing intervention or used home health visits as an outcome measure for a nursing intervention. Therefore, all of the studies (Martens and Mellor 1997; Miller et al. 1996; Brooten, Knapp et al. 1996; Brooten, Naylor et al. 1996) demonstrated links between home health visits and nursing care in nonacute care settings. However, none of the studies tested or confirmed the validity, reliability, sensitivity, or responsiveness of home health visits as an indicator for utilization. One of the studies (Brooten, Naylor et al. 1996) showed the generalizability of a home health intervention for reducing readmissions in seven high-risk, high-volume, and high-cost patient groups. These studies used home health visits in different ways (as part of the intervention and as part of an outcome), so it is difficult to assess the overall ability of nursing interventions to impact home health visits, and thus use home health visits as a link to utilization of services.

Number/Appropriateness of Subacute/Long-Term Care Stays

Two of the studies (Miller et al. 1996; Martens and Mellor 1997) reported on the number/appropriateness of subacute or long-term care (LTC) facility stays as a measure of utilization that is sensitive to the efficacy of nursing interventions. Both studies showed links to nursing care and care in nonacute practice settings. Additionally, both studies supported the responsiveness of LTC utilization to nursing interventions. Generalizability, validity, reliability, and sensitivity of the indicator, however, were not tested nor demonstrated in any of the studies. This indicator is relatively easy to measure.

Number of Minutes per Visit

Three studies were included in the analysis of the number of minutes per visit as an indicator for utilization (Brooten, Knapp et al. 1996; Naylor et al. 1994; Weinberger et al. 1996). All of these studies showed links to nursing and nursing in settings other than acute care. The Naylor et al. and Weinberger et al. studies further demonstrated responsiveness and generalizability of the indicator for measuring utilization in nursing interventions. None of the studies demonstrated validity, reliability, or sensitivity of the indicator. Tools used to measure minutes per visit, however, can be cumbersome for nursing staff because they generally involve a spreadsheet in which nurses enter the amount of time spent either electronically or in hand-written notes.

There is a lot of research to support the scientific merit of the analyzed indicators of utilization of services; however, studies could not be found that tested the validity, sensitivity, or responsiveness of the indicators in this area. Because of the nature of these indicators, they can be assumed to be valid, responsive, and sensitive measures of utilization. Given well-functioning patient electronic record and data systems, these indicators can be easily measured and tailored to capture the impact of the availability or quality of nursing care on utilization of services.

Client/Patient Satisfaction 5

Client satisfaction was defined as the client's perceived satisfaction with various aspects of their nursing care experience, with emphasis on care received in nonacute care settings and the perception of being well cared for by nursing personnel. The identified indicators included satisfaction with nursing care in general, care management, treatment regimen, access to care, and communication. Achievement of client expectations was identified as a potential nursing-sensitive quality indicator; however, there was no evidence in the research-based literature reviewed to support the use of this indicator as a measure of client satisfaction. Therefore, no further analysis was conducted on this indicator.

Satisfaction with Quality of Care Rendered/ Overall Satisfaction with Care

Ten studies measured client/patient satisfaction with the quality of nursing care or overall satisfaction with the care clients/patients received. Eight of the studies (Baradell 1995; Jacox et al. 1997; Lowry et al. 1997; Ludwig-Behmer et al. 1993; Ketefian et al. 1997; Paykel et al. 1982; Ross et al. 1995; Ware and Hays 1988) validated the tools used to measure patient satisfaction or the use of satisfaction with quality of care rendered as an indicator of patient satisfaction. Four of the five studies also determined the reliability of the satisfaction tools. The Lowry and Paykel studies demonstrated not only the reliability but also the sensitivity and responsiveness of this indication. Reliability was also determined by Graveley and Littlefield (1992). Two studies—Graveley and Littlefield's as well that of Rhee and Dermyer (1995)—demonstrated the responsiveness of this indicator. Nine of the studies (all but Ware and Hays) linked patient satisfaction with quality of care rendered directly to nursing care, and seven were specific to nursing care in the nonacute care setting (Baradell; Graveley and Littlefield; Lowry et al.; Paykel et al.; Ketefian et al.; Ross et al.; Ware and Hays). The generalizability of this indicator is evident from the settings, patient demographic characteristics, and patient medical conditions represented in the combined study groups. However, it was particularly apparent in both the Ketefian and the Jacox studies. The tools that measured patient satisfaction with quality of care rendered included patient self-report and mail-in surveys as well as telephone surveys. There is a relatively large amount of literature available on this topic, which would aid in developing a survey and implementation procedures for a tool to measure satisfaction with quality of nursing care rendered.

Satisfaction with Access, Availability, and Timeliness of Care

Five studies measured satisfaction with access, availability, and timeliness of care (Graveley and Littlefield 1992; Rhee and Dermyer 1995; Ross et al. 1995; Safran et al. 1994; Ware and Hays 1988). Three studies validated the tools used to measure client/patient satisfaction with access (Ross, Safran, and Ware and Hays), and another study (Graveley and Littlefield) determined the reliability of the indicator. None of the studies demonstrated sensitivity of the indicator, but three studies (Graveley and Littlefield, Rhee and Dermyer, and Safran et al.) demonstrated the responsiveness and generalizability of the indicator to assess satisfaction with a nursing intervention as compared to other interventions. Ware and Hays also demonstrated the generalizability of patient satisfaction with access measures. All but the Ware and Hays and Safran studies were directly related to nursing care interventions, and all but the Rhee and Dermyer study were conducted in nonacute care settings. (See previous indicator for Quality of Care Rendered for discussion of the ease of measurement.)

Satisfaction with Communication

Four studies supported satisfaction with communication as a measure of overall patient satisfaction. (Ludwig-Behmer et al. 1993; Ketefian et al. 1997; Paykel et al. 1982; Rhee and Dermyer 1995). Two of the studies (Ludwig-Behmer et al. 1993, and Ketefian et al. 1997) assessed the validity of tools to measure client/patient satisfaction with caregiver communication, and another study, Paykel et al., established a link between satisfaction with communication and overall patient satisfaction. The Ketefian study further demonstrated reliability, and the Paykel study demonstrated not only the reliability but also sensitivity and responsiveness of this indicator. The Rhee and Dermyer (1995) study also demonstrated responsiveness of the tool for measuring nursing care as compared to physician care in the emergency room. All of the studies specifically measured satisfaction with the communication of nurses but not other professional groups; however, the Ketefian study measured nursing communication in ambulatory as well as inpatient settings and the Paykel study was conducted in settings other than acute care. As with the indicator for satisfaction with quality of care rendered, the Ketefian study supported the generalizability of the tool used to measure satisfaction with caregiver communication in this study. (See previous indicator for Quality of Care Rendered for a discussion of the ease of measurement.)

Staff Mix

Two studies demonstrated satisfaction with various staff mix models. Graveley and Littlefield (1992) assessed satisfaction of three models for delivering prenatal care to low-risk mothers, including a physician-based model; a mixed-staff model, including physician, nurse practitioner, registered nurses, and nurses aids; and a nurse-based model. This assessment found that the patients receiving the nurse-based model of care had the highest level of satisfaction with their care. Rhee and Dermyer assessed overall satisfaction of members who were seen by a nurse practitioner and compared it with those seen by physicians in an emergency department and found no significant differences in satisfaction between the two groups. The Rhee study supported the validity of staffing mix as an indicator of patient satisfaction. The Graveley study supported the reliability, and the Rhee study supported the responsiveness of this indicator. The Graveley study was the only one to assess nursing care in the nonacute care setting. Generalizability was supported in the Rhee study but was not very well substantiated. (See previous indicator with Quality of Care Rendered for a discussion of the ease of measurement.)

Satisfaction with Treatment Regimens and Satisfaction with Transitions Across Treatment Settings

Ware and Hayes (1988) provided some measurement of satisfaction with treatment regimens and satisfaction with transitions across treatment settings. Validity, reliability, and generalizability were demonstrated for these patient satisfaction indicators but not specifically for nursing. Sensitivity and responsiveness were unfounded from this article alone. The survey instrument, a mail-in instrument, used two different response formats. The survey tool and the procedures for implementing the tool were highlighted in the article and were fairly easy to replicate.

The state of the art in measuring client/patient satisfaction is such that the degree of quality in which rigid scientific standards are met is questionable. Therefore, the analysis of the scientific merit of the indicators in this area must be qualified by this acknowledged limitation. Several of the analyzed indicators were demonstrated to be of acceptable scientific merit; however, more research is needed on the satisfaction with staff mix and satisfaction with treatment regimen and transitions across treatment settings. Due to the nature of these indicators, the methods and tools for measuring them can be tailored to measure the impact of the availability and/or quality of nursing care. The many proven methods for measuring these indicators ranged from quick and easy to time-consuming and very burdensome to any or all parties.

Risk Reduction 6

Risk reduction was defined as behaviors that were adopted by patients to reduce their risk of becoming ill or developing complications, or furthering the progression of their disease or illness. Risk-reduction behaviors involved specific health promotion and disease prevention activities that were conveyed by the nurse to the patient.

Compliance with Medication/Treatment Plan

Five studies related to patient compliance with medication and/or treatment plan (Anderson et al. 1997; Barry 1993; Graham et al. 1993; Erickson and Swain 1990; Proos et al. 1992). Three of the studies validated the compliance indicator for risk reduction (Anderson et al., Graham et al., and Erickson et al.). Only the Anderson study verified the reliability and sensitivity of this indicator. Four of the studies (Anderson, Barry, Erickson, and Proos) demonstrated responsiveness (that is, differences between treatment and control groups). All of the studies demonstrated a link to nursing care, but only three had links to non-acute care settings. Generalizability of the compliance indicator across populations may be inferred from the variety of patients on whom these studies were conducted (that is, cancer patients, diabetics, and hypertensives). Some limitations of these studies included small sample sizes and lack of statistically significant differences between treatment and control groups.

Healthful Lifestyle: Smoking Cessation and Blood Pressure Reduction

Three studies were supportive of healthful lifestyle as an indicator of risk reduction. Two were related to smoking cessation (DeBusk et al. 1994 and Taylor et al. 1990), and one was related to blood pressure reduction (Erickson and Swain 1990). All of the studies found smoking cessation and blood pressure control to be responsive to nursing interventions. However, only Erickson and Swain firmly supported the validity of the indicator for reducing risk of acute myocardial infarction. The DeBusk study supported validity but was not fully realized (that is, there appeared to be favorable trends between smoking cessation and reinfarction rates, but the differences were not statistically significant). All of the studies demonstrated clear links to nursing care and to care delivered in non-acute settings. However, none of the studies specifically tested the reliability or sensitivity of the indicators.

Exercise/Rehabilitation Regimen

Three studies supported exercise/rehabilitation regimens linked to a patient's ability to reduce risk of illness or complications of illness. All three provided some support for the validity as an indicator for risk reduction (DeBusk et al. 1994; McCloskey and Bulechek 1995; Wagner et al. 1994). All but one (McCloskey and Bulechek) demonstrated responsiveness of risk factors to nursing interventions, but none of the studies supported reliability or sensitivity of the indicator. Exercise regimens were administered to persons with AMI and older persons at risk for falling, which lent some support for the generalizability of the indicator. Further studies, however, would need to be done to confirm generalizability. The tools used to measure this indicator consisted of self-report surveys that were fairly easy to administer and inexpensive.

Weight Loss/Control, Appropriate Dietary Intake

Two studies supported weight loss control or appropriate dietary intake as an indicator for risk reduction (DeBusk et al. 1994 and McCloskey and Bulechek. 1995). McCloskey and Bulechek, in particular, validated weight loss interventions for risk reduction, and the DeBusk study lent some support. DeBusk only demonstrated responsiveness of weight loss/dietary indicator to nursing interventions. None of the studies tested reliability or sensitivity. Both studies showed clear links to nursing care, but only DeBusk showed a clear link to care in non-acute settings. Additionally, there was not enough evidence from these studies to support generalizability. One of the main limitations of the studies was that the McCloskey and Bulechek study was based on nursing opinions and not clinical evidence. The tools used to measure this indicator ranged from those that were quick, inexpensive, and readily available (that is, weighing patient) to those that were more costly and time-consuming (that is, measuring LDL levels).

While there was some support for the scientific merit of each of the indicators in this area, all of them require additional research to establish their scientific merit. A wide range of proven tools and methods for measuring these indicators exists; however, the link between the quality or availability of nursing care with these indicators may be difficult to establish.

Increase in Protective Factors 7

Increase in protective factors was defined as behaviors by the client or their caregivers that help protect the client from injury and complications associated with their illness or its treatment. These behaviors often were *indirectly* related to nursing care in that they may have involved a nurse referral to a third party, such as support groups or the poison control number. These behaviors may be those of the patient and/or caregiver and generally involve patients actively seeking assistance with the behavior. Insufficient evidence was found to support the use of number of support groups used by patient, and types of things patient receives assistance with as indicators of increase in protective factors. Therefore, no further analyses were conducted on these indicators.

Existence/Frequency of Primary Caregiver Involvement

Three studies related to the existence/frequency of caregiver involvement. All of the studies (Olds and Kitzman 1990; Anderson et al. 1997; Mittelman et al. 1996) supported the notion that increase in caregiver involvement is a valid indicator for increase in protective factors of an ill patient. The Anderson study, however, was the only study that demonstrated reliability of caregiver involvement (parents) with diabetic patients (children). Anderson and Mittelman together supported the responsiveness of the caregiver involvement indicator in that subjects who underwent treatment to increase involvement of caregivers had better outcomes than those in control groups. Sensitivity was mildly supported by the Anderson article in that varying degrees of the intervention had varying degrees of effect on blood glucose levels, but this needs further testing to substantiate the findings. All of the articles were linked to nursing and to healthcare delivery in nonacute care settings. From the range of patients on whom these studies were conducted (mothers and children, parents of diabetic children, spouse-caregivers of patients with Alzheimer disease), it may be inferred that this indicator is generalizable as well. Anderson described how caregiver involvement was assessed. The study involved nursing staff asking a series of questions about parental involvement in diabetes management. It is assumed that most measures of caregiver involvement would involve administering questionnaires to patients to ascertain the level of involvement. Problems with questionnaire administration, including mail-in survey response rates and nursing staff-administered survey costliness, challenges the use of surveys to measure caregiver involvement.

Injury/Falls Prevention

Seven studies supported injury and falls prevention as an indicator for increase in protective factors (Coenen et al. 1995; Kitzman et al. 1997; Olds et al. 1995; Olds et al. 1997; Olds and Kitzman 1990; Lange 1996; Wagner et al. 1994). Five of the studies (Kitzman et al.; Olds et al. 1995; Olds et al. 1997; Olds and Kitzman; Wagner et al.) demonstrated the validity and responsiveness of injury/falls prevention programs as an indicator for increase in patient protective factors. In addition, Kitzman et al., Olds et al. (1997), and Olds et al. (1995) demonstrated reliability or sensitivity of the indicator. Additionally, all of the studies demonstrated a link to nursing and to practice in nonacute care settings. Generalizability of the indicator may be evidenced by the groups included in the studies (that is, preventing injuries among children and preventing falls in the elderly). Measuring falls and injuries, as noted in these studies and in studies on domestic violence and child abuse, was sometimes difficult. Obtaining reliable numbers for the number of falls or other injuries that may have resulted from abuse or neglect was sometimes contaminated by the desire of patients/caregivers to not report the injury or fall and also by patient/caregiver recall bias.

Equipment Management

One study (Pfaff et al. 1997) assessed equipment management as an indicator for increase in protective factors. In this study, validity and reliability of the indicator were demonstrated, but sensitivity and responsiveness were not. Pfaff's intervention was applicable to care in nonacute care settings. More testing needs to be done to ascertain the generalizability, establish a link to nursing care, and confirm reliability of this indictor for increasing protective factors. The Pfaff study compared two methods for measuring management of medical equipment used in the home, both of which required nursing staff assessment on-site but were not time-consuming or difficult to use.

Use of Recommended Support Groups

A study conducted by Mittelman et al. (1996) ascertained whether the use of recommended support groups was a good indicator for increasing protective factors. This study supported validity and responsiveness of using support groups.

Individuals in an intervention group, which made more use of support groups, delayed nursing home admission of their spouses with Alzheimer's disease to a greater extent than did control group subjects. Sensitivity and reliability of this indicator, however, were not supported by this study. Links to nursing and health care in nonacute care settings were apparent from the intervention used in this study. The generalizability of the indicator, however, was not evident from this study. Further investigation is needed to establish generalizability.

While there is some evidence to support scientific merit of these indicators, further research is needed to establish the sensitivity, reliability, responsiveness, and generalizability of many of them. Proven tools and methods for measuring these indicators exist; however, some may not measure the impact of the quality or availability of nursing care as well as others. These measures ranged from being quick and simple to time-consuming and difficult to use.

Satisfaction with Quality of Life

8

Satisfaction with quality of life was defined as satisfaction with overall quality of life, physical and emotional status, social functioning, and role performance, in light of illness or altered health status that may be influenced by nursing care received. Nursing interventions may involve the development of coping skills and behaviors on the part of the client/family. Note that there was considerable overlap between the indicators in this category and the indicators in patient/client/customer satisfaction and level of functioning. Vitality, percent of day spent in meaningful activity, caregiver/family, and coping/burden/stress were identified as potential nursing-sensitive indicators; however, a search of the research-based literature produced little or no scientific evidence to support the use of these indicators as a measure of patient quality of life. Therefore, no further analyses were conducted on these indicators.

Patient Comfort

Four studies demonstrated some support for patient comfort as an indicator for patient satisfaction with quality of life. Three of the studies (McCloskey and Bulechek 1995; Miakowski and Dibble 1995; Wyatt et al. 1996) demonstrated validity of patient comfort tools, but only the Wyatt study demonstrated reliability of patient comfort as an indicator for satisfaction with quality of life. One of the studies (Peruselli et al. 1997) showed some support, albeit weak, for the sensitivity of the indicator; two studies (Peruselli et al. and Miakowski) confirmed responsiveness. Peruselli et al. and McCloskey and Bulechek showed that patient comfort was linked to nursing care, but only weak links were established with practice in nonacute care settings. Generalizability was not supported by nor was it directly tested in any of the studies, but the combination of the study groups does show weak support for generalizability.

Self-efficacy

All six studies (Baas et al. 1997; Bertero et al. 1997; Grady et al. 1994; McCloskey and Bulechek 1995; Szabo et al. 1997; Wallhagen and Brod 1997) demonstrated the validity of using self-efficacy as an indicator for satisfaction with quality of life. Three of the studies (Baas et al., Grady et al., and Wallhagen and Brod) further demonstrated reliability and responsiveness of self-efficacy indicators. The use of self-efficacy as an indicator in evaluating interventions has been studied across a variety of patient age groups and clinical conditions. It was inferred that results may be generalizable. Only McCloskey and Bulechek showed a clear link to nursing care. None of the studies demonstrated the sensitivity of this indicator, and two studies (McCloskey and Bulechek 1995; Baas et al. 1997) established a weak link to nonacute care nursing. Some of the limitations of the studies included the fact that some (such as Bertero) had small sample sizes, and several studies noted the limitation of not having made a direct link to nursing.

Patient Coping/Burden/Stress

Five studies analyzed patient coping/burden/stress as an indicator for patient satisfaction with quality of life. All of the studies (Keckeisen and Nyamathi 1990; Kuiper and Nyamathi 1991; McCloskey and Bulechek 1995; Grady et al. 1995 Lok 1996) demonstrated validity of this indicator. The studies by Grady et al., Lok, and Keckeisen and Nyamathi also demonstrated reliability of the indicator. Only Grady demonstrated responsiveness. None of the studies demonstrated sensitivity, and only a weak link was made between the indicator and nonacute care nursing (McCloskey and Bulechek 1995; Grady et al.1994). The generalizability of the patient coping indicator may be inferred because each study tested subjects with a different clinical condition, but generalizability was not directly tested in these studies. Limitations of these studies include the lack of a direct link to nursing care and nonacute care settings.

Satisfaction with Social Functioning

Six studies supported the idea that satisfaction with social functioning is related to satisfaction with quality of life. All six studies (Baradell 1995; Bertero et al. 1997; Grady et al. 1995; Ferrell et al. 1989; Lok 1996; Wyatt et al. 1996) demonstrated the validity of social functioning as an indicator of satisfaction with quality of life. Five studies (all but Bertero) supported the reliability of this indicator. However, only Grady demonstrated responsiveness; none of the studies demonstrated sensitivity. Overall generalizability and links between satisfaction with social functioning indicators and nursing practice in nonacute care settings were weak in all but the Baradell study.

Satisfaction with Role Performance

This indicator is closely related to the previous indicator (satisfaction with social functioning), so it is not surprising that four of the six articles from social functioning were also used in support of satisfaction with role performance. The Baradell, Bertero, Grady, and Lok studies demonstrated the validity of using indicators of satisfaction with role performance to measure overall satisfaction with quality of life. Grady and Lok also demonstrated reliability, and Grady demonstrated responsiveness of the satisfaction with role performance indicators. None of the studies, however, showed support for sensitivity or generalizability, and only the Baradell study could be directly linked to nursing care and the nonacute care setting.

Although several articles demonstrated scientific merit of the indicators for this area, further research is needed to support the link to nursing care and generalizability across nonacute care settings. Numerous valid and reliable tools and methods for measuring these indicators exist, and they can be tailored to measure the impact of nursing care; however, they range from simple to very difficult and from quick and easy to very time-consuming to administer.

APPENDIX

A

Nursing Quality Indicators for Settings Other Than Acute Care

Checklist of Indicators and Associated References

This checklist (Table A-1) was used to record two factors:

- achievement of the criterion used to evaluate the scientific merit of the indicators, and
- moderately supported linkages to the criteria that were made in the studies.

The criteria upon which the scientific merit of the indicators was evaluated included the following, each of which is reflected in the columns of the table in this appendix:

- *Availability or quality*—There is an established link to the availability or quality of nursing care: sensitivity to nursing interventions was used as a proxy for this criterion.
- *Nonacute settings*—There is an established link to settings other than acute care.
- *Validity*—There is an established link between the indicator and the ANA-identified area with which it corresponds (such as the indicator predicts the outcome of interest).
- *Reliability*—Any of the following:
  - *Test–retest reliability*—The indicator yields the same results under repeated trials.
  - *Inter-rater reliability*—Different people reviewing the same material have the same results.
  - *Internal consistency*—All of the items of a scale or multi-item measure work together.
- *Sensitivity*—The extent to which the amount of change can be detected and measured. (such as a small but clinically important change can be documented over time).
- *Responsiveness*—There is a change in response to specific nursing interventions or nursing structure.
- *Generalizable*—The indicator has a demonstrated link to a variety of clinical conditions.

TABLE A-1

Indicator	Availability or quality	Nonacute settings	Validity	Reliability	Sensitivity	Responsiveness	Generalizable	References
Change in Symptom Severity:								
Symptom Management/ Relief (pain management/ physical comfort-degree of pain)	■	■	■	■	■	■	■	McCloskey and Bulechek (1995); Peruselli et al. (1997); Rosenthal et al. (1992); Smith et al. (1994); Stucki et al. (1996); Coenen et al. (1995); Vines et al. (1996).
Symptom Management/ Relief (fluid and electrolyte status)	■	■	■	■	■	■	■	McCloskey and Bulechek (1995); Rosenthal et al. (1992); Visalli (1997); Coenen et al. (1995); Rantz et al. (1997).
Symptom Management/ Relief (skin integrity)	■	■	■	■	■	■		McCloskey and Bulechek (1995); Rosenthal et al. (1992); Rantz et al. (1997).
Symptom Management/ Relief (respiratory status)	■	■	■	■	■	■	■	McCloskey and Bulechek (1995); Peruselli et al. (1997); Rosenthal et al. (1992).
Symptom Management/ Relief (nutrition/oral status; includes nausea/vomiting)	■	■	■	■	■	■	■	Graham et al. (1993); McCloskey and Bulechek (1995); Peruselli et al. (1997); Rosenthal et al. (1992); Smith et al. (1994); Rantz et al. (1997).
Frequency/Duration/Intensity of Symptoms (percentage of time spent in improved/ worsened state)	■	■	■	■	■	■	■	Peruselli et al. (1997); Rosenthal et al. (1992); Stucki et al. (1996).
Symptom Management/ Relief (continence)	■	■	■	■	■	■		McCloskey and Bulechek (1995); Rosenthal et al. (1992).
Symptom Management/ Relief (cognition/sensory deficits/ orientation)	■	■	■	■	■	■		Brietbart (1997); McCloskey and Bulechek (1995); Rosenthal et al. (1992, Baradell (1995); Campbell (1992).
Level of Functioning:								
ADLs/IADLs	■	●	■	■	■	■	■	Ottenbacher et al. (1994); Peruselli et al. (1997); Whittle and Goldenberg (1996).
Physical Functioning (exercise tolerance, ambulation, mobility, and transferring)	■	■	■	■	■	■	■	Gortner and Jenkins (1990); McCloskey and Bulechek (1995); Stucki et al. (1996); Whittle and Goldenberg (1996).

KEY TO TABLE:

■ = Strongly demonstrated in literature ● = Moderately supported in literature

TABLE A-1 (*Continued*)

Indicator	Availability or quality	Nonacute settings	Validity	Reliability	Sensitivity	Responsiveness	Generalizable	References
Psychological/neuro/ cognitive functioning	■	■	■	■	■	■		Brietbart et al. (1997); McCloskey et al. (1995); Peruselli et al. (1997); Baradell (1995); Abraham and Reel 1992).
Psychosocial Functioning (emotional/behavioral/ social interaction)	■	■	■	■	■	■	■	Smits et al. (1992); Stucki et al. (1996); Whittle and Goldenberg (1996); Baradell (1995).
Participation in healthcare management (medications and treatment)	■							McCloskey and Bulechek (1995); Vines et al. (1996).
Role Performance	■							Baradell (1995).
Maintenance/Improvement of functioning	■							Peruselli et al. (1997);
Strength of Therapeutic Alliance:								
Coordination of care processes/continuity of care	■	■	■	■		■	■	Brooten et al. (1986); Burns et al. (1996); Naylor, Brooten et al. (1994).
Communication: consistency, timeliness, and style	■	■	■	■	■	■	■	Baradell (1995); Brown (1992); Luborsky et al. (1983); Barnard et al. (1988).
Patient/family involvement in care planning/decision-making	■	■	■		■	■	■	Brooten et al. (1986); Brown (1992); Olds and Kitzman (1990); Szabo et al. (1997); Barnard et al. (1988).
Trust between patient and providers								
Comprehensiveness of care								
Integration of care								
Accuracy of information								
Utilization of Services:								
Number/appropriateness of clinic visits	■	■	■	■	■	■	■	Burns et al. (1996); Miller et al. (1996); Weinberger et al. (1996); Kitzman et al. (1997); Olds et al. (1995).
Number/appropriateness of emergency room visits	■	■	■	■	■	■	■	Brooten et al. (1996b); Burns et al. (1996); Miller et al. (1996); Kitzman et al. (1995); Olds et al. (1995).

KEY TO TABLE

■ = Strongly demonstrated in literature ● = Moderately supported in literature

TABLE A-1 ***(Continued)***

Indicator	Availability or quality	Nonacute settings	Validity	Reliability	Sensitivity	Responsiveness	Generalizable	References
Readmission rates	■	■				■	■	Brooten et al. (1986); Brooten et al. (1996b); Martens and Mellor (1997); Naylor, Brooten et al. (1994); Weinberger et al. (1996).
Number/appropriateness of home health visits	■	■					■	Martens and Mellor (1997); Miller et al. (1996); Brooten et al. (1996a); Brooten et al. (1996b).
Subacute/long-term care stay	■	■				■	■	Miller et al. (1996); Martens and Mellor (1997);
Number of minutes per visit	■	■				■	■	Brooten et al. (1996a); Naylor, Brooten et al. (1994); Weinberger et al. (1996).
Ambulatory-sensitive admission rates								
Number of visits per episode of care								
Client/Patient Satisfaction:								
Satisfaction with quality of care rendered	■	■	■	■	■	■	■	Jacox et al. (1997); Ludwig-Behmer et al. (1993); Graveley and Littlefield (1992); Ketefian et al. (1997); Ware and Hays (1988); Ross et al. (1995); Rhee and Dermyer (1994); Baradell (1995); Lowry et al. (1997); Paykel et al. (1982).
Satisfaction with access to/availability/timeliness of care (e.g., appointment wait times, on-call responsiveness, timeliness of referrals etc.)	■	■	■	■		■	■	Ross et al. (1995); Rhee and Dermyer (1994); Safran et al. (1994); Gravely and Littlefield (1992); Ware and Hays (1988).
Satisfaction with communication	■	■	■	■	●	■	■	Ketefian et al. (1997); Ludwig-Behmer et al. (1993); Rhee and Dermyer (1994); Paykel et al. (1982).
Satisfaction with staff mix	■	●	●	●		●	●	Graveley and Littlefield (1992); Rhee and Dermyer (1995)

KEY TO TABLE

■ = Strongly demonstrated in literature ● = Moderately supported in literature

TABLE A-1 (*Continued*)

Indicator	Availability or quality	Nonacute settings	Validity	Reliability	Sensitivity	Responsiveness	Generalizable	References
Satisfaction with care management/treatment regimen/transition across treatment settings		●	●	●			●	Ware and Hays (1988
Achievement of patient expectations								
Risk Reduction:								
Compliance with medication/treatment plan	■	■	■	●	●	■		Anderson et al. (1997); Barry (1993); Proos et al. (1992); Erickson and Swain (1990); Graham et al. (1993).
Healthful lifestyle (e.g., health screening, smoking cessation, alcohol/drug cessation, motor vehicle safety)	■	■	●			■		DeBusk et al. (1994); Erickson and Swain (1990); Taylor (1990.
Follows exercise/rehabilitation regimen	■	■	■			■	●	DeBusk et al. (1994); McCloskey et al. (1995); Wagner et al. (1994).
Weight control/loss-appropriate dietary intake	■	■	■			■	●	DeBusk et al. (1994); McCloskey et al. (1995).
Increase in Protective Factors:								
Existence/frequency of involvement of a primary caregiver	■	■	■	●	●	■	●	Anderson (1997); Mittelman et al. (1996); Olds and Kitzman (1990).
Injury/falls prevention	■	■	■		■	■	●	Olds and Kitzman (1990); Lange (1996); Wagner et al. (1994); Coenen et al. (1995); Kitzman et al. (1997); Olds et al. (1995); Olds et al. (1997).
Equipment management	●	■	●	●		■	●	Pfaff et al. (1997).
Use of available/recommended support groups	■	■	●			●	●	Mittelman et al. (1996).
Number of supports used by the patient								
Types of things patient receives assistance with								

KEY TO TABLE

■ = Strongly demonstrated in literature ● = Moderately supported in literature

TABLE A-1 ***(Continued)***

Indicator	Availability or quality	Nonacute settings	Validity	Reliability	Sensitivity	Responsiveness	Generalizable	References
Satisfaction With Quality of Life:								
Patient Comfort	■	●	■	■	●	■	●	McCloskey et al. (1995); Miakowski and Dibble (1995); Peruselli et al. (1997); Wyatt et al. (1996).
Self-efficacy	●	●	■	■		■	■	Baas et al. (1997); Bertero et al. (1997); Grady et al. (1994); McCloskey et al. (1995); Szabo et al. (1997); Wallhagen et al. (1997).
Patient coping/burden/stress	●	●	■	■		●	■	Grady et al. (1994); Keckeisen and Nyamathi (1990); Kuiper and Nyamathi (1991); Lok (1996); McCloskey et al. (1995).
Satisfaction with social functioning	■	●	■	■		●	●	Bertero et al. (1997); Grady et al. (1995); Ferrell et al. (1989); Lok (1996); Wyatt et al. (1996); Baradell (1995).
Satisfaction with role performance	■	●	■	■		●	●	Bertero et al. (1997); Grady et al. (1994); Lok (1996); Baradell (1995).
Caregiver/family coping/burden/stress	■	●						Baradell (1995).
Vitality								
Percentage of day spent in meaningful activity								

KEY TO TABLE

■ = Strongly demonstrated in literature ● = Moderately supported in literature

APPENDIX B

Annotated Bibliography

For this annotated bibliography, articles were abstracted by obtaining the following information:

- Purpose of the study
- Description of the sample
- Methods and data analysis
- Time frame of the study
- Findings (including the statistical significance, if noted)
- Relationship between the indicator and nursing care
- Relevance of the findings to settings other than acute care
- Any study limitations

The references reviewed and annotated for this bibliography are listed starting on the next page. The annotations start on page 41, grouped by the following areas of interest, which are described in the Executive Summary. (See Appendix C for a list of the references used to identify these identifiers.)

1. Changes in symptom severity
2. Level of functioning
3. Strength of the therapeutic alliance
4. Utilization of services
5. Patient/client satisfaction
6. Risk reduction (environmental and behavioral)
7. Increase in protective factors
8. Satisfaction with quality of life

Since some of the indicators appear under more than one category, there was some overlap in the indicators identified for each of the areas, and some of the articles will be referenced in multiple places.

Annotated References

The following references were reviewed and annotated for this bibliography.

Abraham, I.L., and S.J. Reel (1992). Cognitive nursing interventions with long-term care residents: effects on neurocognitive dimensions. *Archives of Psychiatric Nursing* VI (6): 356–65.

Anderson, B., J. Ho, J. Brackett, D. Finkelstein, and L. Laffel (1997). Parental involvement in diabetes management tasks: relationships to blood glucose monitoring adherence and metabolic control in young adolescents with insulin-dependent diabetes mellitus. *The Journal of Pediatrics* 130(2): 257–65.

Baas, L.S., J.A. Fontana, and G. Bhat (1997). Relationship between self-care resources and the quality of life of persons with heart failure: a comparison of treatment groups. *Progress in Cardiovascular Nursing* 12(1): 25–38.

Baradell, J.G. (1995). Clinical outcomes and satisfaction of patients of clinical nurse specialists in psychiatric–mental health nursing. *Archives of Psychiatric Nursing* IX(5): 240–50.

Barnard, K.E., D. Margyary, G. Sumner, C.L. Booth, S.K. Mitchell, and S. Spieker (1988). Preventing parenting alterations for women with low social support. *Psychiatry* 51: 248–53.

Barry, K. (1993). Patient self-medication: An innovative approach to medication teaching. *Journal of Nursing Care Quality* 8(1): 75–82.

Bertero, C., B.E. Eriksson, and A.C. Ek (1997). A substantive theory of quality of life of adults with chronic leukemia. *International Journal of Nursing Studies* 34(1): 9–16.

Brietbart, W., K. Barry, A. Roth, M. Smith, K. Cohen, and S. Passik (1997). The memorial delirium assessment scale. *Journal of Pain and Symptom Management* 13(2): 128–37.

Brooten, D., H. Knapp, L. Borucki, B. Jacobsen, S. Finkler, L. Arnold, and M. Mennuti (1996a). Early discharge and home care after unplanned cesarean birth: Nursing care time. *Journal of Obstetrics, Gynecology, and Neonatal Nursing* September, 25(7): 595–600.

Brooten, D., S. Kumar, L.P. Brown, P. Butts, S.A. Finkler, S. Bakewell-Sachs, A. Gibbons, and M. Delivoria-Papadopoulos (1986). A randomized clinical trial of early hospital discharge and home follow-up of very low birthweight infants. *The New England Journal of Medicine* 315(15):934–9.

Brooten, D., M. Naylor, L. Brown, R. York, A. Hollingsworth, S. Cohen, M. Roncoli, and B. Jacobsen (1996b). Profile of postdischarge rehospital izations and acute care visits for seven patient groups. *Public Health Nursing* 13(2): 128–34.

Brown, S.J. (1992). Tailoring nursing care to the individual client: empirical challenge of a theoretical concept. *Research in Nursing and Health* 15: 39–46.

Burns, L.R., G.S. Lamb, and D.R. Wholey (1996). Impact of integrated community nursing services on hospital utilization and a Medicare risk plan. *Inquiry* 33(1): 30–41.

Coenen, A., P. Ryan, J. Sutton, E.C. Devine, H.H. Werley, and S. Kelber (1995). Use of the Nursing Minimum Data Set to describe nursing interventions for select nursing diagnoses and related factors in an acute care setting. *Nursing Diagnosis* 6(3): 108–14.

Debusk, R.F., N. H. Miller, H. R. Puerko, C.A. Dennis, R.J. Thomas, H.T. Lew, W.E. Berger, R.S. Heller, J.G. Rompf, D. Gee, H.C. Kraemer, A. Bandura, G. Ghandour, M.Clark, R.V. Shah, L. Fisher, and C.B. Taylor (1994). A case-management system for coronary risk factor modification after acute myocardial infarction. *Annals of Internal Medicine* 120(9): 721–9.

Erickson, H., and M.A. Swain (1990). Mobilizing self-care resources: a nursing intervention for hypertension. *Issues in Mental Health Nursing* 11: 217–35.

Ferrell, B.R, C. Wisdom, and C. Wenzl (1989). Quality of life as an outcome variable in the management of cancer pain. *Cancer* 63: 2321–7.

Gortner, S.R., and L.S. Jenkins (1990). Self-efficacy and activity level following cardiac surgery. *Journal of Advanced. Nursing* 15(10): 1132–8.

Grady, K.L., A. Jalowiec, C. White-Williams, R. Pifarre, J.K. Kirklin, R.C. Bourge, and M.R. Costanzo (1995). Predictors of quality of life in patients with advanced heart failure awaiting transplantation. *Journal of Heart and Lung Transplantation* 14(1): 2–10.

Graham, K.M., D.A. Pecoraro, M. Ventura, C.C. Meyer (1993). Reducing the incidence of stomatitis using a quality assessment and improvement approach. *Cancer Nursing* 16(2): 117–22.

Graveley, E.A., and J.H. Littlefield (1992). A cost-effectiveness analysis of three staffing models for the delivery of low-risk prenatal care. *American Journal of Public Health* 82(2): 180–4.

Jacox, A.K., B.R. Bausell, and D.M. Mahrenholz (1997). Patient satisfaction with nursing care in hospitals. *Outcomes Management in Nursing Practice* 1(1): 20–8.

Keckeisen, M.E., and A.M. Nyamathi (1990). Coping and adjustment to illness in the acute myocardial infarction patient. *Journal of Cardiovascular Nursing* 5(1): 25–33.

Ketefian, S., R. Redman, M.G. Nash, E.L. Bogue (1997). Inpatient and ambulatory patient satisfaction with nursing care. *Quality Management in Health Care* 5(4): 66–75.

Kitzman, H., D.L. Olds, C.R. Henderson, C. Hanks, R. Cole, R. Tatelbaum, K.M. McConnochie, K. Sidora, D.W. Luckey, D. Shaver, K. Engelhardt, D. James, and K. Barnard (1997). Effect of prenatal and infancy home visitation by nurses on pregnancy outcomes, childhood injuries, and repeated childbearing. *Journal of the American Medical Association* 278(8): 644–53.

Kuiper, R., and A.M. Nyamathi (1991). Stressors and coping strategies of patients with automatic implantable cardioverter defibrillators. *Journal of Cardiovascular Nursing* 5(3): 65–76.

Luborsky, L., P. Crits-Christoph, L. Alexander, M. Margolis, and M. Cohen (1983). Two helping alliance methods for predicting outcomes of psychotherapy: counting signs vs. a global rating method. *Journal of Nervous and Mental Disease* 171(8): 480–91.

Lange, M (1996). The challenge of fall prevention in home care: A review of the literature. *Home Healthcare Nurse* 14(3): 198–206.

Lok, P. (1996). Stressors, coping mechanisms, and quality of life among dialysis patients in Australia. *Journal of Advanced Nursing* 23: 873–81.

Lowry, L., J. Saeger, and S. Barnett (1997). Client Satisfaction with prenatal care and pregnancy outcomes. *Outcomes Management for Nursing Practice* 1(1): 29–35.

Ludwig-Behmer, P., C.J. Ryan, N.J. Johnson, K.A. Hennessy, M.C. Gattuso, R. Epsom, and K.T. Czurylo (1993). Using patient perceptions to improve quality care. *Journal of Nursing Care Quality* 7(2): 42–51.

Martens, K.H., and S.D. Mellor (1997). A study of the relationship between home care services and hospital readmissions of patients with congestive heart failure. *Home Healthcare Nurse* 15(2): 123–9.

McCloskey, J., and G. Bulechek (1995).Validation and coding of the NIC taxonomy structure. *Image: Journal of Nursing Scholarship* 27(1): 43–9.

Miakowski, C., and S.L. Dibble (1995). The problem of pain in outpatients with breast cancer. *Oncology Nursing Forum* 22(2): 791–7.

Miller, L.L., M.C. Hornbrook, P.G. Archbold, B.J. Stewart (1996). Development of use and cost measures in a nursing intervention for family caregivers and frail elderly patients. *Research in Nursing and Health* 19: 273–85.

Mittelman, M.S., S.H. Ferris, E. Shulman, G. Steinberg, and B. Levin (1994). A family intervention to delay nursing home placement of patients with Alzheimer disease: a randomized controlled trial. *Journal of the American Medical Association*. 276(21): 1725–31.

Naylor, M., D. Brooten, R. Jones, R. Lavizzo-Mourey, M. Mezey, and M. Pauly (1994). Comprehensive discharge planning for the hospitalized elderly: a randomized clinical trial. *Annals of Internal Medicine* 120(12): 999–1006.

Olds, D.L., J. Eckenrode, C.R. Henderson, H. Kitzman, J. Powers, R. Cole, K. Sidora, P. Morris, L.M. Pettitt, and D. Luckey (1997). Long-term effects of home visitation on maternal life course and child abuse and neglect: fifteen year follow-up of a randomized trial. *Journal of the American Medical Association* 278(8): 637–43.

Olds, D., C.R. Henderson, H. Kitzman, and R. Cole (1995). Effects of prenatal and infancy nursing home visitation on surveillance of child maltreatment. *Pediatrics* 95(3): 365–72.

Olds, D.L., and H. Kitzman (1990). Can home visitation improve the health of women and children at environmental risk? *Pediatrics* 86(1): 108–16.

Ottenbacher, K.J., W.C. Mann, C.V. Granger, M. Tomita, D. Hurren, and B. Charvat (1994). Inter-rater agreement and stability of functional assessment in the community-based elderly. *Archives of Physical and Medical Rehabilitation* 65: 1297–301.

Peruselli, C., E. Paci, T. Francheschi, T. Legori, and F. Mannucci (1997). Outcome evaluation in a home palliative care service. *Journal of Pain and Symptom Management* 13(3): 158–65.

Pfaff, K.M., L.E. Johnson, P.J. Savage, and J.R. Kues (1997). Evaluation of an assessment tool for equipment management (ATEM) of home oxygen concentrators. *Respiratory Care* 42(6): 611–16.

Proos, M., P. Reiley, J. Eagan, S. Stengrevics, J. Castile, and D. Arian (1992). A study of the effects of self-medication on patients' knowledge of and compliance with their medication regimen. *Journal of Nursing Care Quality* Suppl: 18–26.

Rantz, M.J., L. Popejoy, D.R. Mehr, M. Zwygart-Stauffacher, L.L. Hicks, V.G. Grando, V.S. Conn, R. Porter, J. Scott, and M. Maas (1997). Verifying nursing home care quality using minimum data set quality indicators and other quality measures. *Journal of Nursing Care Quality* 12(2): 54–62.

Rhee, K.J., and A.L. Dermyer (1995). Patient satisfaction with a nurse practitioner in a university emergency service. *Annals of Emergency Medicine* 26(2): 130–2.

Rosenthal, G.E., E.J. Halloran, M. Kiley, C. Pinkley, C.S. Landefeld, and the nurses of University Hospitals of Cleveland (1992). Development and validation of the nursing severity index: a new method for measuring severity of illness using nursing diagnoses. *Medical Care* 30(12): 1127–41.

Ross, C.K., C.A. Steward, and J.M. Sinacore (1995). A comparative study of seven measures of patient satisfaction. *Medical Care* 33(4): 392–406.

Safran, D.G., A.R. Tarlov, and W.H. Rogers (1994). Primary care performance in fee-for-service and prepaid health care systems: results from the medical outcomes study. *The Journal of the American Medical Association* 271(20): 1579–86.

Smith, M.C., J.K. Holcombe, and E. Stullenbarger (1994). A meta-analysis of intervention effectiveness for symptom management in oncology nursing research. *Oncology Nursing Forum* 21(7): 1201–9.

Smits M., and C. Kee (1992). Correlates of self-care among the independent elderly: self-concept affects well-being. *Journal of Gerontological Nursing* 18(9): 13–18.

Stucki, G., L. Daltroy, M.H. Liang, S.J. Lipson, A.H. Fossel, and J.N. Katz (1996). Measurement properties of a self-administered outcome measure in lumbar spinal stenosis. *Spine* 21(7): 796–803.

Szabo, E., H. Moody, T. Hamilton, C. Ang, C. Kovithavongs, and C. Kjellstrand (1997). Choice of treatment improves quality of life: a study on patients undergoing dialysis. *Archives of Internal Medicine* 157: 1352–6.

Taylor, O.B., N. Houston-Miller, J.D. Killen, and R.F. DeBusk (1990). Smoking cessation after acute myocardial infarction: effects of a nurse-managed intervention. *Annals of Internal Medicine* 113(2): 118–23.

Vines, S.W., A. Cox, L. Nicoll, and S. Garrett (1996). Effects of a multimodal pain rehabilitation program: a pilot study. *Rehabilitation Nursing* 21(1): 25–30, 40.

Visalli, H. (1997). Developing a best practice model for care of patients with polydipsia. *Journal of Nursing Care Quality* 12(1): 53–62.

Wagner, E.H., A.Z. LaCroix, L. Grothaus, S.G. Leveille, J.A. Hecht, K. Artz, K. Odle, and D.M. Buchner (1994). Preventing disability and falls in older adults: a population-based randomized trial. *American Journal of Public Health* 84(11): 1800–6.

Wallhagen, M.I., and M. Brod (1997). Perceived control and well-being in Parkinson's disease. *Western Journal o f Nursing Research* 19(1): 11–31.

Ware, J.E., and R.D. Hays (1988). Method for measuring patient satisfaction with specific medical encounters. *Medical Care* 26(4): 393–402.

Weinberger, M., E.Z. Oddone, and W.G. Henderson (1996). Does increased access to primary care reduce hospital readmissions? *The New England Journal of Medicine* 334(22): 1441–7.

Whittle, H., and D. Goldenberg (1996). Functional health status and instrumental activities of daily living performance in noninstitutionalized elderly people. *Journal of Advanced Nursing* 23: 220–7.

Wyatt, G., M.E. Kurtz, L.L. Friedman, B. Given, and C.W. Given (1996). Preliminary testing of the Long-Term Quality of Life (LTQL) instrument for female cancer survivors. *Journal of Nursing Measurement* 4(2): 153–70.

1. Changes in Symptom Severity

Baradell, J.G. (1995). Clinical outcomes and satisfaction of patients of clinical nurse specialists in psychiatric–mental health nursing. *Archives of Psychiatric Nursing* IX(5): 240–50.

This study determined whether patients who have terminated from psychotherapy with a clinical nurse specialist (CNS) report improvement in clinical symptoms, improvement in quality of life, and satisfaction with the relationship and services provided by the CNS. The study also determined what led the patient to select a CNS for psychotherapy and whether or not there is a positive relationship between clinical outcomes and levels of satisfaction. An ex post facto design was used to evaluate the clinical outcomes and level of satisfaction from patients who had terminated psychotherapy with a CNS over a one-year time frame. Data were collected through a mail survey. The study involved 235 patients of six certified CNSs who had terminated therapy between January 1, 1993, and December 31, 1993. Demographic and clinical data were collected using a CNS data collection form. The data were separated into the two categories, and the clinical data were identified by a four-digit code number. Clinical data included start and termination dates, the number of treatments, the treatment modality used, and the patient's Global Assessment Function (GAF) on initiation of and termination from treatment. The patient's survey instruments included Profile of Mood States-Short Form (POM-SF), Quality of Life (QOL), and Patient Satisfaction Survey (PSS). Patients were asked to complete the POM-SF for how they felt when they started therapy and how they have felt since they terminated therapy. The patients were sent a survey by their therapist in July 1994; those who had not responded were sent a follow-up reminder postcard three weeks later. There were 100 usable returns, yielding a response rate of 45 percent. Overall, patients reported excellent clinical outcomes and a very high level of satisfaction with the psychotherapy provided by the CNSs. Improvement of clinical symptoms reported was significant, and there was a significant improvement in quality of life. Ninety-five percent of participants rated the services provided by the CNSs as "excellent," "very good," or "good." The results indicated a significant positive correlation between patients' reports of improvement in clinical symptoms and satisfaction with the care provided ($p = .0002$), patient improvement in QOL and overall satisfaction with the care provided ($p = .0001$), and improvement in clinical symptoms and overall satisfaction with interpersonal relationships ($p = .0088$).

The results of this study demonstrated the relationship between symptom management/relief cognition, psychological/neurological/cognitive functioning, communication, satisfaction with social functioning, satisfaction with role functioning, satisfaction with family coping, and satisfaction with quality of care rendered and the quality or availability of nursing care.

Brietbart, W., K. Barry, A. Roth, M. Smith, K. Cohen, and S. Passik (1997). The memorial delirium assessment scale. *Journal of Pain and Symptom Management* 13(2): 128–37.

The two studies described in this article assessed the reliability and validity of a measure of delirium severity, the Memorial Delirium Assessment Scale (MDAS). The first study involved thirty-three patients: seventeen had met the DSM III-R/DSM IV criteria for delirium, eight had met diagnostic criteria for another cognitive impairment disorder, and eight had noncognitive psychiatric disorders. The patients with nondelirium cognitive disorders and noncognitive psychiatric disorders acted as controls. Multiple raters jointly administered the MDAS to these patients. The results indicated high levels of inter-rater reliability for the MDAS (0.92) and the individual MDAS items (0.64–0.99). There were also high levels of internal consistency (coefficient alpha = 0.91). Mean MDAS ratings differed significantly between the study patients and the controls ($p = .002$). The second study compared MDAS ratings of fifty-one medically hospitalized delirious patients with cancer and AIDS to other measures of delirium, including the Delirium Rating Scale and clinician's ratings of delirium severity, and other measures of cognitive functioning, including the Mini-Mental State Examination. A different clinician applied each of the scales to all of the patients. The results demonstrated a high correlation between the MDAS scores and all of the other ratings (Delirium Rating Scale: $r = .88$, $p < .0001$; the Mini-Mental State Examination: $r = .91$, $p < .0001$; and clinician's global ratings of delirium and severity: $r = .89$, $p < .0001$).

The findings suggest a relationship between delirium and cognitive impairment. In addition, they demonstrate that a variety of cognitive assessment tools can be used to determine the existence and severity of cognitive symptoms and that there are tools, such as the MDAS, that demonstrate both validity and inter-rater reliability. A limitation of this study is that it did not test nursing interventions to influence delirium or cognitive impairment.

Coenen, A., P. Ryan, J. Sutton, E.C. Devine, H.H. Werley, and S. Kelber (1995). Use of the Nursing Minimum Data Set to describe nursing interventions for select nursing diagnoses and related factors in an acute care setting. *Nursing Diagnosis* 6(3): 108–14.

This study described the prevalence of nursing interventions across six nursing diagnoses: pain, potential for injury, anxiety, decreased cardiac output, potential for infection, and knowledge deficit. The setting for the study was a public hospital that shared services with six other facilities comprising a Midwestern Regional Health Care Center. During 1991, 13,135 patients were admitted to the hospital, and the hospital had a computerized Nursing Information System (NIS) that linked the elements of the Nursing Minimum Data Set. The NANDA classification system was used in the NIS. The nursing interventions were classified by code into sixteen categories and linked to the nursing diagnoses. The sample was taken from the patients with one or more of the six identified nursing diagnoses. The prevalence of nursing intervention categories was examined for each of the diagnoses. Across all six diagnoses, teaching was the most frequent intervention, and it was selected 34 percent of the time.

This study demonstrated the validity of symptom management/relief for pain, and fluid and electrolyte status as indicators of change in symptom severity. In addition, it established the link between symptom management/relief for pain, fluid and electrolyte status, and injury prevention and the quality or availability of nursing care.

Campbell, J.M.(1992). Treating depression in well older adults. *Issues in Mental Health Nursing* 13: 19–29.

This study determined if nurses could identify maladaptive depression in well, older adults and whether nursing intervention strategies made a significant difference in levels of depression in the well elderly. A nonprobability sample was selected from residents of two city-owned and two privately owned high-rise apartments for low-income, well, elderly persons. The group identified as depressed consisted of eighty women and twenty-three men aged 64 to 82 years. All of the subjects were diagnosed with nonsuicidal, nonpsychotic depression based on the criteria of the *Diagnostic and Statistical Manual of Mental Disorder, 3rd edition* (DSM-III-R). The nurses on staff in the four buildings were asked to use the DSM-III-R to identify fifty residents per building who were, in their judgment, depressed. One hundred three residents who met the established criteria agreed to participate in the study. Subjects were assigned to three groups stratified by random sample according to gender, which resulted in equal gender distributions in each group. Group 1 received planned nursing interventions per a protocol that was based on cognitive therapy techniques, Group 2 received no intervention, and Group 3 received group classes and practice on crafts, but no specific treatment from nurses to rule out the Hawthorne effect. Study participants were informed of the study's purpose, the time frame, expectations, and the nurses' role. Nurses were given training on the use of the DSM-III-R, and the protocols planned for nursing intervention strategies. Subjects in the intervention group received individual therapy from an assigned nurse for eight weeks, with two one-hour interventions per week. The subjects were seen privately in common rooms of the housing units. One hundred twelve individuals were identified as depressed, instead of the originally planned 200 participants. Of the 112, 103 were identified as being depressed by scoring at least in the moderately depressed range. The Zung Self-Rating Depression Scale (SRDS) was used to validate the ability of the nurses to identify depressed individuals. Their results were validated with 92 percent accuracy. At the conclusion of the nursing intervention, all of the individuals in the experimental group achieved Zung SRDS scores indicating mild or no depression, while the individuals in the nonintervention groups showed no changes from the original scores that demonstrated moderate to severe depression. The difference between the scores before and after the nursing intervention were statistically significant ($t = 3.83, p > 1$). There was also a significant difference between the median scores of the subjects in the craft group and in the experimental group (Mann-Whitney U = 27; $p > .05$).

The results of this study support the validity, sensitivity, and responsiveness of management/relief of cognitive symptoms as an indicator of change in symptom severity. Furthermore, the results of the study demonstrated a link between the quality or availability of nursing interventions in a nonacute care setting and the severity of patients' cognitive symptoms.

Graham, K.M., D.A. Pecoraro, M. Ventura, and C.C. Meyer (1993). Reducing the incidence of stomatitis using a quality assessment and improvement approach. *Cancer Nursing* 16(2): 117–22.

The findings show a trend toward a decreased percentage of patients with stomatitis over the more than two-year period in which data were collected from July 1989 to September 1991. The findings of this data support the validity of patient compliance with medication regimen as an indicator for risk reduction and the validity of management of symptoms of oral/nutritional status as an indicator for change in symptom severity. In addition, it verified the responsiveness of oral/nutritional status to nursing interventions. The limitations of this study are that tests of statistical significance were not conducted, and the reliability and generalizability of these findings has not been determined. (See the section on Risk Reduction for a description of this study.)

McCloskey, J., and G. Bulechek (1995). Validation and coding of the NIC taxonomy structure. *Image: Journal of Nursing Scholarship* 27(1): 43–9.

This study validated the Nursing Interventions Classification (NIC) taxonomy structure. The NIC is a three-tiered structure having 6 domains, 26 classes, and 357 interventions. Previously, a rigorous research approach was used to develop the taxonomy. To validate the NIC, a questionnaire to assess the meaningfulness of the classes and domains was distributed in May 1993 to a sample of nurses who belonged to three interest groups in the Midwest Nursing Research Society (MNRS). Of the 295 members of the interest groups of theory development, qualitative methods, and nursing diagnosis who were polled, the 161 MNRS members who responded that they were willing to assist were sent the questionnaires. One hundred thirty (81 percent) responded. Of the 130 surveys returned, 121 were used for the study and the other 9 were returned late or did not include all of the necessary information. Each participant was mailed a copy of the NIC and a survey. They were asked to rate each domain and each call of the NIC according to the following five criteria: clarity, homogeneity, inclusiveness, mutual exclusiveness, and theory neutrality. The ratings were entered into a mainframe computer and the Statistical Analysis System (SAS) was used to determine the number of respondents and frequencies for each criteria for each class and domain. Seventy-seven percent of respondents rated the domains as either quite characteristic or very characteristic on all criteria, and 88 percent of the respondents rated the classes as either quite characteristic or very characteristic on all criteria. The criteria of theory neutral and mutual exclusiveness received the highest ratings and the criterion of inclusiveness received the lowest ratings. The Physiological Complex domain received the highest ratings, and the Health System domain received the lowest ratings. The respondents also submitted written comments that were reviewed by one of six subgroups of the research team and summarized in a report of the groups' findings and conclusions. The summaries were then reviewed by leaders of the research team and incorporated into the taxonomy. The taxonomy was validated.

The results of this study support the face validity of the relationship between the quality or availability of nursing care and activity and exercise management, elimination management, immobility management, nutrition support, physical comfort promotion, self-care facilitation, electrolyte and acid-base management, drug management, neurologic management, perioperative care, respiratory management, skin and wound management, thermoregulation, tissue perfusion management, behavior therapy, cognitive therapy, communication enhancement, coping assistance, patient education, psychological comfort promotion, crisis management, risk management, childbearing care, life-span care, health system mediation, health system management, information management, crisis management, and risk management (abuse, delirium, delusion, dementia, environmental management, fall prevention, health screening, immunization administration, infection control, pressure ulcer prevention, radiation therapy management, and seizure management). The weakness of this study is that it is based on professional opinions and does not involve the clinical testing of the impact of nursing interventions on any of these areas.

Peruselli, C., Francheschi P. Eugenio, T. Legori, and F. Mannucci (1997). Outcome evaluation in a home palliative care service. *Journal of Pain and Symptom Management* 113(3): 158–65.

This study described the patient's quality of life at the beginning and throughout the process of palliative care at home and defined some potential indicators of palliative care outcomes with the aim of assessing the quality of home care as provided by a palliative care unit. The study included 106 advanced cancer patients treated by a Pain Therapy and Palliative Care hospital unit from July 1992 to April 1993. Of the patients included in the study, thirty-three were treated in the outpatient clinic and seventy-three were treated at home during the last few weeks of life. Fifty-five of the seventy-three patients treated at home were treated for at least ten days; these patients were included in the study. The duration of the home care period had a median of twenty-nine days. For each patient enrolled in the study, the following data were collected: a patient form compiled during the first visit included personal data, initial diagnosis, diagnosis date, referral source, reference doctor, previous treatments, and degree of patient awareness; a form compiled during weekly staff meetings reported the number of visits made, nursing diagnoses, and any significant changes in therapy; and a weekly evaluation of the degree of physical self-sufficiency was made by the nurse using three Katz activity of daily living (ADL) tests. A weekly evaluation of the degree of symptom distress was performed using the symptom distress scale (SDS) developed by McCorkle and Young. The SDS analyzed the distress level of patients linked to thirteen different symptoms (intensity and frequency of pain, intensity and frequency of nausea, appetite, insomnia, bowel pattern, respiration, coughing, fatigue, concentration, appearance, and mood) using Likert-type scales, with scores ranging from 1 to 5. To compare scores for SDS total and subscales, summary measures were obtained for each patient considering the score at the beginning of palliative home care, the mean score after the second week of home care, and before the last two weeks before death, and the highest score over the last two weeks of life. If the difference between the second and first scores was negative, an indication of lower distress, this was considered to be related to the intervention of the palliative care unit. A positive value was a sign of increasing distress before death. The standard deviation of the second score was considered an indicator of the stability of the patient's conditions after the first visit and before the last two weeks of life. The differences between the second and first scores and the last and second scores were weighted for the standard deviation of the second score, obtaining two new responsiveness indexes. Ninety-five percent confidence intervals of each of the three scores were estimated using standard errors. The difference between the second and first scores (–2.1; $p = .08$) suggested an improvement of symptom control after the initiation of home nursing care. The difference between the last and second scores (4.2; $p = .002$) suggested that distress is worsening (as expected) as the patient approached death.

The largest improvement in symptoms secondary to quality nursing care was seen in the pain, functional, and psychological subscales. These results demonstrated that home nursing care can decrease the severity of pain and the psychological and functional symptoms experienced by patients. The results also showed that the severity of these symptoms changes and is measurable over time. These results should be generalizable to other nonacute care settings.

Rantz, M.J., L. Popejoy, D.R. Mehr, M. Zwygart-Stauffacher, L.L. Hicks, V.G. Grando, V.S. Conn, R. Porter, J. Scott, and M. Maas (1997). Verifying nursing home care quality using minimum data set quality indicators and other quality measures. *Journal of Nursing Care Quality* 12(2): 54–62.

This study independently verified the accuracy of the quality indicators (QI) derived from the minimum data set (MDS) using four different methods: structured participative observation, the QI Observation Scoring Instrument, Independent Observable Indicators of Quality Instrument, and survey citations. This was done by analyzing the range of quality outcome performance of nursing homes in a statewide MDS database to independently verify observed care quality with MDS QI scores, evaluating the utility of qualitative data collection and scoring instruments for the care processes and outcomes measured by MDS QIs, and evaluating the sensitivity of an independent, quantitative measure of observable care quality developed by the research team. Included in the MDS is information about each resident's cognitive abilities, functional abilities, presence of depression, disease profile, and rehabilitation/restorative treatment. The study analyzed fourteen of the thirty existing QIs that were determined to have sufficient variation among facilities, were related to well-documented quality problems in nursing homes, represented diverse aspects of quality care, and were amenable to clinical practice interventions. These included the prevalence of injury, falls, problem behavior towards others, incontinence, incontinence without a toileting plan, indwelling catheters, fecal impaction, weight loss, bedfast residents, daily physical restraints, little or no activity, stage 1–4 pressure ulcers, and insulin-dependent diabetes with no foot care. Using 1994–1995 MDS data, nursing homes that performed particularly well and particularly poorly on the Health Care Financing Administration (HCFA) sponsored Nursing Home Case Mix and Quality Demonstration (NHCMQ). Thirty-five nursing homes in Missouri were identified as performing well, and 124 homes were identified as performing poorly. A research nurse who had no knowledge of the QI performance results of the homes contacted them and asked them to participate in a quality of care study. Ten homes agreed to participate: five identified as performing well and five identified as performing poorly. A qualitative data collection instrument and a detailed data collection procedure were designed and followed by the research nurse and research team. A second instrument was constructed to score observations of care delivery for each MDS QI. A third instrument was tested during the observation periods. Using participant observation methods and a qualitative QI observation instrument, data were collected during daylong, on-site observation of care delivery for each of the ten nursing homes. Descriptive analysis of the scores revealed a strong association between the MDS QI scores, the QI Observation Instrument scores, the participant observation findings, Indicators of Quality scores, and the mean number of citations received by a nursing home for 1994–1995. Homes with good quality outcomes generally had more registered professional nurses actively involved in carte. These homes also had good care processes, such as focused ambulation/mobility programs to encourage mobility, toileting programs to promote continence, and nutritional programs to assure that residents' nutritional needs were met. The RNs in good quality homes were not nurses solely hired to complete the MDS process, but assessed residents reported as having problems, took responsibility for communication with physicians, and directed the care and treatment plans for residents. They also served in educational and supportive roles to the non-RN nursing staff. The number of decubitis ulcers stage II and above, prevalence of weight loss, incontinence, and restraints were fewer in homes with good quality scores than in those with poor quality scores.

The study results suggested that the symptoms of skin integrity, nutrition and oral status, and fluid and electrolyte status are valid, responsive, and sensitive indicators of the quality of nursing care. In addition, the results suggested that there is a relationship between the education and training of the nursing staff and quality of care delivered in nursing homes. The scientific weaknesses of the study included that it only involved a sample of ten nursing homes, the study used a purposive rather than a random sample of nursing homes, the instruments/tools used for the study had not undergone previous testing. In addition, the study was primarily descriptive in nature.

Rosenthal, G.E., E.J. Halloran, M. Kiley C. Pinkley, C.S. Landefeld, and the nurses of University Hospitals of Cleveland (1992). Development and validation of the nursing severity index: a new method for measuring severity of illness using nursing diagnoses. *Medical Care* 30(12): 1127–41.

This study determined whether a symptom severity index used by nursing was a valid indicator of severity of the patient's illness. The study design was a retrospective cohort study with two phases: development and testing. In the development phase, data for 13,183 patients admitted to an academic medical center in 1985 and 1986 were used. In the testing phase, data for 7,302 patients admitted to the same medical center between 1987 and 1988 were used. Demographic and clinical data for the patients were obtained from the hospital database. The nursing severity index includes thirty-four nursing diagnoses in the areas of physiologic alterations, physical and social functioning, cognition, nutrition, mood, and social support. The index includes diagnoses related to many different areas, including nutrition, continence, fluid balance and status, respiratory status, cognitive functioning, skin integrity, and pain. Both the number of admission nursing diagnoses ($p < .001$) and the Nursing Severity Index ($p < .001$) were strongly related to in hospital patient mortality.

The results of this study indicated that symptom severity and changes in symptom severity are measurable by nurses. In addition, nutrition, continence, fluid balance and status, respiratory status, cognitive functioning, skin integrity, and pain are valid, reliable, responsive, and sensitive indicators of symptom severity. Some of the limitations of this study are that it did not directly link changes in symptom severity to the availability or quality of nursing care, and it was conducted in an acute care setting.

Smith, M.C., J.K. Holcombe, and E. Stullenbarger (1994). A meta-analysis of intervention effectiveness for symptom management in oncology nursing research. *Oncology Nursing Forum* 21(7): 1201–9.

This study assessed the effectiveness of nursing symptom management in oncology patients. The research design included an integrative research review and meta-analysis. Experimental studies were identified and coded by four oncology nurse specialists, and findings were transformed into effect size. Effect sizes were combined into overall effect for the twenty-eight studies, and the effects were clustered by symptoms, interventions, and outcomes. For the twenty-eight symptom management studies, the weighted average effect was $d = 0.47$. The 95-percent confidence interval ranged from 0.31 to 0.61. The statistical significance was $p = 5.17 \times 10^{-12}$

with wide variability of effect ($\chi^2 = 66.574$, df = 27; $p = 3.41 \times 10^{-5}$) and success rate improved from 39 percent to 62 percent for subjects in the treatment group. The research team concluded that nursing interventions were effective for managing nausea and vomiting, pain, anxiety, alopecia, and side effects from chemotherapy.

The results indicate that the symptom severity indicators of nutritional status and pain are sensitive to the quality or availability of nursing care.

Stucki, G., L. Daltroy, M.H. Liang, S.J. Lipson, A.H. Fossel, and J.N. Katz (1996). Measurement properties of a self-administered outcome measure in lumbar spinal stenosis. *Spine* 21(7): 796–803.

This study tested the measurement properties and validity of a short, self-administered questionnaire on symptom severity, physical functional status, and patient satisfaction. The items for the questionnaire were chosen using a literature review and consultation from an expert panel. The scales were tested in an ongoing prospective, observational study of patients undergoing surgery at three teaching hospitals. Consecutive patients referred to the five surgeons involved in the study for evaluation of spinal stenosis were eligible for the study. Demographic and disease-related inclusion criteria were used. Patients unable to complete questionnaires because of cognitive or language difficulties were excluded from the study. Patients were assessed prior to surgery and six months postoperatively. A random sample of patients was e-mailed two identical questionnaires two weeks apart to assess test–retest reliability. At baseline, neuromuscular signs, radiographic findings, and demographic characteristics were abstracted from medical records using standard coding forms. Comorbidity was assessed with the Cumulative Illness Rating Scale. At baseline and six months postoperatively, data on symptom severity, physical functioning, a visual analog scale measure of pain, the Sickness Impact Profile, depression, and sociodemographic characteristics were collected using mailed questionnaires. At six months postoperatively, the patients were also asked to complete a patient-satisfaction questionnaire. The questionnaire includes three scales with seven questions on symptom severity, five on physical functioning, and six on satisfaction. The internal consistency of the scales was assessed with Cronbach's coefficient alpha on cross-sectional data from 193 patients prior to surgery. The test–retest reliability was tested on data collected from a random sample of twenty-three patients using Spearman's rank correlation coefficient. The responsiveness was assessed on the six-month follow-up data from 130 patients using the standardized response mean. The test–retest reliability of the scales was 0.94 for symptom severity, 0.91 for the pain domain, 0.81 for the neuroischemic domain, 0.94 for the physical functioning scale, and 0.96 for the patient-satisfaction scale. The internal consistency was 0.64 for the symptom severity scale, 0.73 for the pain domain, 0.63 for the symptom severity domain, 0.82 for the physical functioning scale, and 0.92 for the patient satisfaction scale. The responsiveness was 0.96 for the symptom severity scale, 1.0 for the pain domain, 0.56 for the neuroischemic domain, and 1.07 for the physical functioning scale. The assessment of the patient's capacity to ambulate was strongly associated with physical functioning ($r = .47$; CI, 0.36–0.56). Patients with gait disturbances had significantly worse functional scores than those without gait disturbance (2.9 versus 2.6, $p < .01$). The symptom severity scale was strongly correlated with pain measured on a visual analog scale ($r = .52$, CI, 0.41–0.62). The pain domain showed correlations with both physical and psychological functioning aspects of the SIP ($r = .34$ and .31, respectively; CI 0.121–0.46 and 0.18–0.40, respectively). The satisfaction scale was highly correlated with the change in symptom severity and a better score in the physical function scale ($r = .66$ and .68, respectively; CI, to 0.73 and 0.75, respectively).

In addition to demonstrating the reproducibility, internal consistency, validity, and responsiveness of the questionnaire, this study demonstrated the validity, reliability, sensitivity, and responsiveness of pain as an indicator of symptom severity, physical functioning, and psychosocial functioning; ambulation as an indicator of physical functioning; and symptom severity and level of functioning as indicators of patient satisfaction. One limitation of this study is that there is no direct link to nursing interventions or nursing practice.

Vines, S.W., A. Cox, L. Nicoll, and S. Garrett (1996). Effects of a Multimodal Pain Rehabilitation Program: A Pilot Study. *Rehabilitation Nursing* 21(1): 25–30, 40.

The purpose of this study was to examine the effects of a multimodal pain rehabilitation program on the pain perceptions, pain medication usage, activity, down time, sleep, and role function status of 23 chronic pain patients. The study was conducted in a freestanding rehabilitation hospital with 80 inpatient beds and an active outpatient program. The multidisciplinary program involved nurses, psychiatrists, psychologists, social workers, physical therapists, occupational therapists, and vocational rehabilitation workers. Enrollment in the program is based on patients having pain for which there is no further medical or surgical interventions and experiencing significant difficulty in performance of activities of daily living (ADLs), or emotional, physical, or social functioning. Exclusion criteria include medical, substance abuse, or psychiatric problems that are not under control. During the 12-month period from July 1992 to June 1993, complete data were obtained from 23 of the 30 patients who participated in the program. All of the patients were white, the majority were female, and the ages ranged from 17 to 78 years of age with a mean of 46 years of age. Medicaid, Medicare, Workers Compensation, or private insurance covered the costs of the program. A numeric verbal analog scale (VAS) measured pain levels. In prior studies, the VAS has been found to be a reliable measure of pain in both adult and adolescent populations. Activity level and sleep disturbances were assessed by asking a series of questions. Questions concerning medication usage were limited to patients' self-reports. Pretest and posttest patient interviews and a retrospective chart review were used to collect data on the variables of interest. After completing the program, patients reported a significant reduction in their pain levels (M = 4.5, SD = 1.9, $t[20] = 10.9$, p, .05), a significant reduction in the number of days with decreased activity (M = 3.5, SD = 1.2, $t[11]$ 9.5, p, .05) a significant decrease in sleep disturbances (SD +1.6, $t[11] = 6.9$, p, .05), a decrease in down time (SD = 4.2), and an increase in the number of hours in role functions (SD = 8.2).

These results demonstrate the validity, responsiveness, and sensitivity of pain as an indicator of symptom severity. The study also demonstrates a correlation between level of comfort and physical functioning. The study demonstrates a relationship between nursing interventions and pain; however, the extent of the impact is not measured. Although this study occurs in two very specialized non-acute care settings, the results appear to be generalizable. A limitation of the study includes the small sample size.

Visalli, H. (1997). Developing a best practice model for care of patients with polydipsia. *Journal of Nursing Care Quality* 12(1): 53–62.

The study revised nursing practice to develop an effective uniform approach to caring for patients with polydipsia. A review of current practice determined that a small group of polydipsia patients required a large amount of one-on-one staff time, and no benefit in their symptom status was realized as a result. Furthermore, there was not a uniform approach for the identification, treatment, and outcomes monitoring of polydipsia patients. A team was assembled to develop a protocol for assessing polydipsia and an associated treatment map. The outcome was the development of a care map using diagnostic procedures and nursing interventions supported in the professional literature and empirical data collected on site. The diagnostic procedures and treatment plan were developed after a retrospective study of three polydipsia patients on Clozaril who were successfully treated and discharged to the community for one year. A six-month pilot study of the protocol has resulted in a number of polydipsia patients being discharged on Clozaril using the treatment map.

The results of this study indicated that fluid status is a valid indicator of symptom severity which is sensitive to the quality and availability of nursing care and is generalizable across nonacute care settings. The limitations of this study are the lack of detailed information about the design, subjects, methodology and data analysis used. The description of the interventions is very detailed, but the description of the pilot study is brief and vague.

2. Level of Functioning

Abraham, I.L., and S.J. Reel (1992). Cognitive nursing interventions with long-term care residents: effects on neurocognitive dimensions. *Archives of Psychiatric Nursing* VI(6): 356–65.

This study determined whether nursing interventions would produce improvements in the cognitive functioning of nursing home residents. The sample consisted of seventy-six older adults residing in seven nursing homes who met sampling criteria specific to subjects' ability to participate in group interventions. Of these subjects, thirty participated in cognitive-behavioral groups, twenty-nine in focused visual imagery groups, and seventeen in education-discussion groups. There were nineteen, fifteen, and eight left in each of the respective groups for the posttreatment data collection. Applying power tables from Kirk, the residual subsample sizes satisfied the requirements for detecting differences. A recently developed but psychometrically strong extension of the Mini-Mental State Exam was used to screen cognitive status and dementia. Three clinical nurse specialists with credentials and experience in respective treatment modalities conducted 24-week group interventions. Four trained interviewers who were unaware of the treatment conditions to which subjects were assigned were randomly assigned to each of the nursing homes. Data were collected according to a preestablished calendar four weeks before interventions, eight and twenty weeks after the initiation of treatment, and four weeks after the conclusion of the interventions. To quantify the change in scores on cognitive parameters for subjects in a given treatment condition, a standardized index was derived. The results demonstrated that there were significant differences in the results achieved with the various interventions ($F(2,36) = 3.91; p = .05$). With main effects for the type of intervention on the Similarities ($F(2, 36) = 3.32; p < 5$), Mental Reversal ($F(2,36) = 3.59; p < .05$), and Writing ($F(2,36) = 3.58; p < 5$) portions of the score. Changes in all but one of the five categories of cognitive performance were identified.

The results of this study supported the validity, sensitivity, and responsiveness of cognitive functioning as an indicator of level of functioning. In addition, the results of this study established a link between the quality or availability of nursing care in nursing homes and level of cognitive functioning. The limitations of this study include the small sample size and the limited information presented about any other cognitive interventions that the subjects were receiving.

Baradell, J.G. (1995). Clinical outcomes and satisfaction of patients of clinical nurse specialists in psychiatric–mental health nursing. *Archives of Psychiatric Nursing* IX(5): 240–50.

The results of this study demonstrated the relationship between symptom management/relief cognition, psychological/neurological/cognitive functioning, communication, satisfaction with social functioning, satisfaction with role functioning, satisfaction with family coping, and satisfaction with quality of care rendered and the quality or availability of nursing care. (See the section on Changes in Symptom Severity for a description of this study.)

Barnard, K.E., D. Margyary, G. Sumner, C.L. Booth, S.K. Mitchell, and S. Spieker (1988). Preventing parenting alterations for women with low social support. *Psychiatry* 51: 248–53.

This study determined whether the development of a therapeutic relationship between pregnant women and their visiting nurse would reduce the experience of social-emotional disturbances and developmental delay by their children. One hundred and thirty-seven pregnant women in their second trimester who lacked social support were recruited from public health clinics in King County, Washington. The participants were randomly assigned to one of two treatment groups that received home visiting nursing care by a consistent caregiver, following a written protocol, with specific goals and objectives. Sixty-eight women received the Mental Health model of treatment. The primary focus of this treatment was on establishing a therapeutic relationship with the client. In this model, the nurse fostered a relationship with the client based on the general theories of Lawrence Brammer: the nurse demonstrated through the nurse-client relationship ways of dealing with interpersonal situations and problem solving, and the client was an active participant in her care. The other sixty-nine participants received treatment according to the Information/Resource model of care. The objective of this model was to provide information, facts, and procedures in a straightforward way. Each woman was visited in her own home throughout her pregnancy and the infant's first year of life. Evaluation data were collected at regular intervals, beginning at the time that the woman started the program and ending when the child was 3 years old. The data were collected using a combination of interviews, observation, and questionnaires. Measures used for evaluating maternal competency included the Beck Depression Inventory (BDI), the Personal Resource Questionnaire, the Community Life Skills Scale, and the Social Skills Scale. Parent-child interaction was evaluated using the Nursing Child Assessment Teaching Scale (NCATS) and the Nursing Child Assessment Feeding Scale (NCAFS). The environment was evaluated using the Home Observation for Measurement of the Environment (HOME). The child's competency was measured using several standardized tests, including the Bayley Developmental Scales, Mastery Motivation tests, the Achenbach Child Behavior Checklist, and the Ainsworth Strange Situation. In addition, detailed data were collected about the frequency, content, and process of the nursing interventions. The nursing acts were defined as monitoring, informing, support, and providing therapy. Ninety-five participants, or 65 percent, of those enrolled in the study were retained throughout the three-year period. The women who dropped out of the study were less socially competent as measured on the project scales of community life skills, social skills, and perceived social support. While 80 percent of the Mental Health model treatment group remained in the study, only 53 percent of the Information/Resources group remained. There were no group differences in pregnancy outcomes and no significant differences between the children in the two groups. The Mental Health group had more nurse contact ($t[127] = 3.84$, $p < .001$), a greater relative frequency of nursing "therapy" acts ($t[131] = 5.90$, $p < .001$), and attained more of the treatment goals ($t[105] = 2.71, p < .01$). The women in the Information/Resource group received a greater relative frequency of the "informing" nursing acts ($t[131] = 5.90$, $p < .01$). The mothers in the Mental Health group demonstrated less depression. Also, more of them who initially scored low in social competencies scored high by the end of the study, they scored higher on the HOME and MCAST tests at the end of the study, and they had a more positive view of their world. Further studies determined that mothers with lower IQ scores (less than 90), using the Quick Test demonstrated more secure attachments and better outcomes in the mothers and children using the Mental Health model. The women with higher IQ scores and their children fared better in the Information/Resource model group.

This study demonstrated that patient/family involvement in care planning/decision-making and tailoring home visiting nurses' communication to the client's needs can improve the client's treatment outcomes by increasing the strength of the therapeutic alliance. The study supported the validity, sensitivity, and responsiveness of patient/family involvement in care planning/decision-making and communication as indicators of the strength of the therapeutic alliance.

McCloskey, J., and G. Bulechek (1995). Validation and coding of the NIC taxonomy structure. *Image: Journal of Nursing Scholarship* 27(1): 43–9.

The results of this study support the face validity of the relationship between the quality or availability of nursing care and activity and exercise management, elimination management, immobility management, nutrition support, physical comfort promotion, self-care facilitation, electrolyte and acid-base management, drug management, neurologic management, perioperative care, respiratory management, skin and wound management, thermoregulation, tissue perfusion management, behavior therapy, cognitive therapy, communication enhancement, coping assistance, patient education, psychological comfort promotion, crisis management, risk management, childbearing care, life-span care, health system mediation, health system management, information management, crisis management, and risk management (abuse, delirium, delusion, dementia, environmental management, fall prevention, health screening, immunization administration, infection control, pressure ulcer prevention, radiation therapy management, and seizure management). The weakness of this study is that it is based on professional opinions and does not involve the clinical testing of the impact of nursing interventions on any of these areas. (See the section on Changes in Symptom Severity for a description of this study.)

Ottenbacher, K.J., W.C. Mann, C.V. Granger, M. Tomita, D. Hurren, and B. Charvat (1994). Inter-rater agreement and stability of functional assessment in the community-based elderly. *Archives of Physical and Medical Rehabilitation* 65: 1297–301.

This study analyzed the inter-rater reliability and test–retest reliability of the Functional Independence Measure and the Instrumental Activities of Daily Living (IADL) from the Multidimensional Assessment of Older Adults. The study involved twenty randomly selected subjects participating in a larger study of consumer needs related to disability and technology. The larger sample included 348 persons more than 60 years of age who were receiving assistance from a human services agency and living in home-based settings in the community. Two experienced raters administered the two instruments over a seven- to ten-day period or a four- to six-week period. Intraclass correlation (ICC) values for inter-rater agreement and stability were computed. They ranged from .90 to .99. The relation between the scores on the two different scales was also examined. The analysis indicated that there was a positive statistical relationship between the items assessed ($r = .085$). The high ICC values indicate the FIM and the IADL measurement of the Multidimensional Functional Assessment of Older Adults provide consistent information across two experienced raters and over time when used with a sample of elderly persons residing in the community.

The results of this study demonstrated the reliability of IADLs as an indicator of functional status and demonstrate the ability to use this indicator across nonacute care settings. The limitations of this study include the lack of a direct link to nursing care, the small sample size of the study population, and the failure to test the link between the validity of IADL score as an indicator of functional status.

Peruselli, C., E. Paci, P. Francheschi, T. Legori, and F. Mannucci (1997). Outcome evaluation in a home palliative care service. *Journal of Pain and Symptom Management* 13(3): 158–65.

The largest improvement in symptoms secondary to quality nursing care was seen in the pain, functional, and psychological subscales. These results demonstrated that home nursing care can decrease the severity of pain and the psychological and functional symptoms experienced by patients. The results also showed that the severity of these symptoms changes and is measurable over time. These results should be generalizable to other nonacute care settings. (See section on Changes in Symptom Severity for a description of this study.)

Smits, M., and C. Kee (1992). Correlates of self-care among the independent elderly: self-concept affects well-being. *Journal of Gerontological Nursing* 18(9): 13–18.

This study was conducted to determine whether there was a significant, positive relationship between self-concept and self-care; whether there were significant differences in self-concept by demographic categories; and whether a significant positive relationship existed between functional health status and self-care. This study included a convenience sample of forty-eight voluntary participants of age 65 or older who were living independently. Ages of the subjects ranged from 65 to 97 years, with a median age of seventy-nine years. Women outnumbered men forty-two to six. About half of the subjects resided in independent retirement complexes, half were participants in senior citizen center activities, and four were contacted through personal referral. Data were collected in the meeting rooms of these settings or in the people's homes. The Tennessee Self-Concept Scale (TSCS) was used to measure self-concept. Self-care was measured through the Exercise of Self-Care Agency Scale (ESCA). Roscow and Breslau's Guttman Health Scale for the Aged was employed to measure functional health. The first hypothesis, posing a relationship between self-concept and self-care, was tested using Pearson's product-moment correlation. Total and subscale scores on the TSCS were each correlated with the score attained on the ESCA. A significant relationship was found between self-care and self-concept and between self-care and the self-concept subscales of social and physical self, self-satisfaction, and behavior, at the .001 level of confidence. The second hypothesis, that there would be differences in self-care scores based on selected demographic characteristics, was not supported. No differences were found using *t*-test procedures in self-care scores. The third hypothesis, that there would be a significant relationship between self-care, self-concept, and functional health status led to mixed results. While a significant correlation to self-concept and functional status was found, a significant relationship between self-care and functional status was not found.

This study validated the correlation between psychosocial status, and functional status and suggests that nurses may improve the functional status of patients by focusing on psychosocial as well as physical interventions. However, the impact of nursing care on the psychosocial functioning of patients was not directly addressed in this study. The results are generalizable across nonacute care settings.

Stucki, G., L. Daltroy, M.H. Liang, S.J. Lipson, A.H. Fossel, and J.N. Katz (1996). Measurement properties of a self-administered outcome measure in lumbar spinal stenosis. *Spine* 21(7): 796–803.

In addition to demonstrating the reproducibility, internal consistency, validity, and responsiveness of the questionnaire, this study demonstrated the validity, reliability, sensitivity, and responsiveness of pain as an indicator of symptom severity, physical functioning, and psychosocial functioning; ambulation as an indicator of physical functioning; and symptom severity and level of functioning as indicators of patient satisfaction. One limitation of this study is that there is no direct link to nursing interventions or nursing practice. (See the section on Change in Symptom Severity for the description of this study.)

Whittle, H., and D. Goldenberg (1996). Functional health status and instrumental activities of daily living performance in noninstitutionalized elderly people. *Journal of Advanced Nursing* 23: 220–7.

This study ascertained whether a relationship existed between elderly people's functional health status and their level of independence in instrumental activities of daily living (IADLs). This study was conducted using a descriptive correlational design. A convenience sample of forty-seven subjects 70 years of age or older, able to understand and respond to written English, and who had noninstitutionalized living arrangements voluntarily participated. The study was conducted in three family practice offices and a geriatric clinic associated with a large teaching hospital. The reported chronic health conditions of the subjects included arthritis, angina, hypertension, and chronic obstructive pulmonary disease. The study subjects completed a demographic questionnaire, the Multidimensional Functional Status Assessment Questionnaire/Instrumental Activities of Daily Living Scale (MFSAQ/IADL), and the Health Status Questionnaire (HSQ). Statistical analysis was performed using the Statistical Package for the Social Sciences (SPSS) program. The relationship between functional health status and performance of the IADLs was tested using inferential statistics using a .05 level of significance for the data analysis. Frequency data obtained from the MFSAQ/IADL scale was used to determine the dependency in each of the IADLs. Lawton's (1985) theoretical model of person-environment interaction provided the conceptual framework for this study. Three functional status variables reached statistical significance in relationship to IADL performance, indicating that they are important indicators of overall health status, and that a decline in any of them could contribute to increased IADL dependency. The number of IADL dependencies reported was significantly associated with physical functioning ($r = .6511$; $p = .001$), social functioning ($r = .5467$; $p = .01$), and health perception ($r = .6107$; $p = .001$).

The results demonstrate that IADL performance is a valid indicator of both physical and social functioning. They also demonstrate the ability to measure differences in functional status. This has significance for nurses with regard to using health promotion and disease management strategies related to the independence of patients, although this article does not demonstrate the effects of nursing care on the performance of IADLs. These findings are generalizable across nonacute care settings.

3. Strength of the Therapeutic Alliance

Brown, S.J. (1992). Tailoring nursing care to the individual client: empirical challenge of a theoretical concept. *Research in Nursing and Health* 15: 39–46.

This study determined the empirical adequacy of one conceptual specification of individualization of care, tailoring, which is a concept in Cox's Interaction Model of Client Health Behavior (IMCHB). The central proposition of Cox's theory is that "health outcome is determined by the fit of the provider reactions to the clients' responses to a health concern, as well as to the clients' physical and socioenvironmental characteristics." Cox interchangeably uses the terms *tailoring*, *fit*, and *matching* to refer to achieving congruence between the actions of the nurse and the unique characteristics of the client. The client-professional interaction element consists of interpersonal actions by which the nurse influences the client and manages the client's clinical condition; all of these actions are accomplished through interpersonal interaction. The IMCHB has previously been tested and both the individuality of the client and the client professional relationship/ interaction were significant determinants of health decisions and subsequent health behavior. According to Cox, the nurse tailors care to the individual client when he takes into account the client's singularity and allows that singularity to determine interactional approaches and plans of intervention. The interpersonal approaches that operationally define tailoring in this study were the following: attending to a client's singularity; discussing client singularity and clinical assessment-management content in association rather than separately; and producing interventions that are explicitly personalized to the individual. Tailoring of care is viewed as a joint endeavor of the nurse and client. This joint interaction proceeds via discourse as the two participants allow their separate perceptions, values, and goals to interact and influence each other. Initially, six encounters between clients who were receiving pregnancy care and a nurse practitioner who was judged to be an expert nurse based on reputation, experience, and education were audiotaped over a two-day period. Although participants consented to audiotaping, none of them knew the purpose of the research. A course-grained listening analysis was conducted on the six tapes to select three encounters with the most surface manifestations of tailoring. Two separate codings of the tapes by the same rater were conducted, separated by a three-week interval, and resulted in selection of the same three tapes. The three clients in the sample were between 20 and 23 years old. The nurse practitioner had been in her role for approximately one year, working part time, and had been in obstetrical nursing for twelve years. The setting was a private practice clinic. Clients alternated visits with a nurse practitioner and an obstetrician, and the longest actual visit was 14.5 minutes. The analysis of the content in relationship to the components of the IMCHB involved coding each segment of the tape using a content coding scheme. The second analysis involved examining stretches of talk to determine the topical focus of each. The analysis of interventions consisted of determining whether the interventions were explicitly personalized to the individual and her circumstances. Inter-rater reliability estimates consisting of unitizing reliability indexes and global interpretive agreement indexes for nominal level measurement were established for each analysis. Unitizing reliability for the analysis of content of the segments was 1.0. The global interpretive agreement was 0.79. Unitizing reliability for the analysis of the topical focus of stretches of talk was 0.91, and the global interpretive agreement was 0.81. Unitizing reliability for the analysis of interventions was 0.89, and global interpretive agreement was 1.00.

Together, the theoretical elements predicted 72 percent, 83 percent, and 79 percent of the content segments of the respective encounters. The findings of these three analyses support the existence of tailoring as an approach to care utilized by this expert nurse in cooperation with clients. This study supports the theory that both communication style and the degree to which care is patient-centered are valid indicators of the strength of the therapeutic alliance. The results appear to be generalizable across settings; however, the small sample size used in this study limits the weight of any conclusions that are drawn from it. In addition, the methods used to measure both communication style and the degree to which nursing care is patient-centered are burdensome for the person evaluating the strength of the therapeutic alliance.

Brooten, D., S. Kumar, L.P. Brown, P. Butts, S.A. Finkler, S. Bakewell-Sachs, A. Gibbons, and M. Delivoria-Papadopoulos (1986). A randomized clinical trial of early hospital discharge and home follow-up of very low birthweight infants. *The New England Journal of Medicine* 315(15): 934–9.

This study was conducted to examine whether it is safe and economical to discharge very low birthweight infants early if they meet certain criteria. Between October 1982 and December 1984, 72 mothers and 79 infants were randomized into control and treatment groups. The control group members had to be clinically stable, feeding well, and weigh approximately 2200 g. Parents received usual instructions from the nursery nurses, but no routine home care was provided. The treatment group infants could be discharged if they weighed less than 2200 g, but they had to meet some stringent criteria to ensure that the infant was doing well and not at risk for complications. The criteria were that the infant was clinically stable, able to feed every four hours, able to maintain body temperature in open crib in room air, had no evidence of serious apnea or bradycardia, the mother or other caretaker demonstrated satisfactory care-taking skills, and the physical home environment and facilities for the care of the infant were adequate. The treatment group received home follow-up care provided by a nurse in the first week and at 1, 9, 12, and 18 months after discharge from the hospital. The nurse was in contact with the parents by telephone at least three times a week for the first two weeks and weekly thereafter for the following eight weeks. Prior to discharge, the nurse met with the parents soon after the infant's birth and at least once a week during the infant's hospitalization. The purpose of the in-hospital visits was to educate the parents about caring for their infant, preparing them for the discharge, and establishing a rapport between the parents and the nurse, all of which provided continuity for parents as the infant was being transferred from the hospital to the home. There were no statistically significant differences between the groups on parent and infant demographic characteristics. The treatment group infants were discharged an average of 11.2 days before the control group infants ($p < .05$) and weighed approximately 200 g less. (This is not statistically significant. The treatment groups also showed trends for lower rehospitalization, acute care visits, and child abuse cases. In addition to the frequent phone calls initiated by the nurses, parents made over 300 telephone calls to the nurses during the follow-up period. The mean charges for initial hospitalization were significantly lower for the treatment group ($47,520) than the control group ($64,940) ($p < .01$, a one-tailed test). In addition, the mean charge for physician services was lower ($p < .01$). The mean cost per infant to provide in-hospital and 18 months of follow-up care (i.e., home care visits, telephone calls, travel time, and nurse time) was $576. On the basis of these findings, the authors concluded that early discharge of very low birthweight infants, using standards identified in the study, is safe, feasible cost-effective, and provides continuity of care.

The study supported the use of the indicators for family involvement in care planning and decision making and coordination of care processes/ continuity of care for the strength of the therapeutic alliance. Additionally, it supports the use of readmission rates as an indicator for utilization. The study was not designed to test the validity or reliability of these indicators, but it does show some weak support for its validity. It also shows that outcomes for infant care are positively impacted by a nursing intervention that took place in a nonacute care setting. Additionally, with the differences between the treatment and control groups, the study demonstrates that the indicators are responsive to nursing care.

Luborsky, L., P. Crits-Christoph, L. Alexander, M. Margolis, and M. Cohen (1983). Two helping alliance methods for predicting outcomes of psychotherapy: counting signs vs. a global rating method. *Journal of Nervous and Mental Disease* 171(8): 480–91.

This study showed the development of methods for measuring helping alliances in psychotherapy. One of the methods is the counting signs method, whereby judges count certain types of patient statements (i.e., signs) that are identified in a manual. There were two broad types of counting signs—those in which the patient experiences the therapist as providing or being capable of providing the help that is needed and those in which the patient experiences treatment as a process of working together with the therapist toward the treatment goals. The other method is a global rating referred to as the helping alliance rating, which is described more fully in other literature but involves inference from a judge who must comprehend the entire sample of the psychotherapy to infer the degree to which the patient experiences a helping alliance. Twenty patients were selected from among 73 in the Penn

Psychotherapy Project to participate in the project, including 10 of the most improved and 10 of the least improved patients. For each patient, there were 4 sessions that judges reviewed, each lasting about 20 minutes long. Manuals for the 2 methods were applied to the 80 sessions by 2 different pairs of independent judges. The judges were clinically experienced and given practice sessions on how to use the manuals. The judges using the counting signs method were from different practice areas (clinical psychology and social work) and different institutions. The judges for the rating method were experienced psychoanalysts who had previously worked together. The results concentrated on the findings from the counting signs method, since the rating method had been tested and reported in earlier literature. The most frequent counting signs reported were those in which the patient feels the therapy is helping and those in which the patient feels changed from the beginning of treatment in ways in which the patient considers to be better. There was moderate inter-rater agreement in the number of signs scored by the judges. Positive items were agreed on particularly well, with correlations ranging from .69 to .82 for the different sessions. The counting signs scores and the rating score were correlated, particularly for the late sessions. The methods also proved to be helpful in predicting outcomes, as they showed statistically significant correlations with rated benefits ($r = .57$, $p < .01$) and first targeted complaint ($r = .59$; $p < .01$). In other words, those who were most improved showed more positive signs and those who were least improved showed more negative signs.

The results show how an indicator for helpful treatment is a valid, reliable, and sensitive measure of the strength of therapeutic alliance. Although this study was not linked to nursing, there was a link to care that takes place in the nonacute care settings. More specifically, the findings can be generalized to patients being treated with psychotherapy in outpatient settings.

Naylor, M., D. Brooten, R. Jones, R. Lavizzo-Mourey, M. Mezey, and M. Pauly (1994). Comprehensive discharge planning for the hospitalized elderly: a randomized clinical trial. *Annals of Internal Medicine* 120(12): 999–1006.

This study examined the effects of a comprehensive discharge planning protocol, designed specifically for the elderly and implemented by nurse specialists, on patient and caregiver outcomes and charges for care. The sample included 272 patients who were 70+ years of age, admitted from their homes to the Hospital of the University of Pennsylvania, were alert and oriented when admitted, able to speak English, and were from selected medical and surgical DRGs for heart conditions. The medical DRGs were congestive heart failure and angina/myocardial infarction; the surgical DRGs were coronary artery bypass graft and cardiac valve replacement. The patients were randomized into treatment and control groups, stratified by medical or surgical DRGs. The control groups received routine discharge planning from the hospital. The treatment groups received the routine discharge plan plus a comprehensive individualized discharge planning protocol developed specifically for elderly patients and implemented by a gerontological clinical nurse specialist. The protocol covered the period from the hospital up to two weeks after discharge. It involved the nurse specialist meeting with the patient and caregiver within 24 to 48 hours of admission, and meeting with the patient every 48 hours thereafter to implement patient and caregiver education, referrals, consultation with health care team members, counseling, and coordination of home services. Additionally, the nurse was available seven days a week by phone during the hospital stay and the two weeks following discharge to answer any questions about the discharge plan. The nurse also initiated a minimum of two phone calls after discharge to monitor patient's progress and intervene as necessary. There were no significant differences on demographic or health status variables between the medical and surgical intervention groups and their corresponding control groups. The mean length of stay and charges for the initial hospital stay were similar for the medical and surgical intervention groups and their corresponding control groups. The mean length of time between the index hospital discharge and readmission for patients in the medical DRGs was 45.6 days for the treatment group and 31.0 days for the control group (p = .12). For surgical DRG patients, the means length of time was 28.9 days for the intervention group and 21.4 days for the control group (p = .34). Within two weeks of discharge for the initial hospitalization, there were more patients in the medical DRG intervention group that were readmitted than patients in the control group (p = .02). No significant differences were reported after two weeks for the surgical DRG groups. Medical and surgical intervention groups were similar in mental status, functional status, perception of health, self-esteem, and affect as measured two weeks after discharge, between 2 and 6 weeks after discharge, and between 6 and 12 weeks after discharge. Mean charges for other health services after discharge were significantly lower for the intervention group ($1,237) than for the control group ($3,613) ($p$ = .06). The study found that nurse specialists had a mean of 4.8 personal visits and telephone contacts with patients and caregivers while patients were hospitalized. During the two-week period after discharge, the nurse specialist had a mean of 2.5 telephone contacts with patients and caregivers. They spent a mean of 3.59 hours on discharge planning during hospitalization and a mean of 46.4 minutes during the two-week follow-up period after discharge.

This study showed weak support for the validity of two indicators in the strength of therapeutic alliance area, including patient/family involvement in care planning and coordination of care processes/continuity of care. It also lent some validity to using a readmission indicator for the area of health service utilization. There was a clear link to nursing care and although the discharge planning protocol was mostly implemented in the acute care setting, there was a weak link to nonacute care in that patients and caregivers could access the nurse after discharge from the hospital. Further, the differences between the treatment and control groups supported the responsiveness of the indicators.

Olds, D.L., and H. Kitzman (1990). Can home visitation improve the health of women and children at environmental risk? *Pediatrics* 86(1): 108–16.

This study demonstrated the validity and responsiveness of home nursing interventions to improve environmental factors influencing maternal and child health, including injury prevention and use of primary caregiver. It also demonstrated the validity and responsiveness of interventions that incorporated strong therapeutic alliances between mothers and families with the home-visiting nurse. As this review noted, additional studies must be conducted using the same models (as those described in the Elmira, Seattle, and Washington, DC, studies) to confirm the reliability of the findings from these studies. (See section on Increase in Protective Factors for a description of this study.)

Szabo, E., H. Moody, T. Hamilton, C. Ang, C. Kovithavongs, and C. Kjellstrand (1997). Choice of treatment improves quality of life: a study on patients undergoing dialysis. *Archives of Internal Medicine* 157: 1352–6.

This study suggests that patient involvement in the treatment plan/strength of the therapeutic alliance is a valid indicator of patient satisfaction with quality of life. A limitation of this study is that it was not directly linked to nursing interventions. However, nurses have the ability to involve patients in their treatment decisions regardless of the setting. (See section on Satisfaction with Quality of Life for a description of this study.)

4. Utilization of Services

Brooten, D., H. Knapp, L. Borucki, B. Jacobsen, S. Finkler, L. Arnold, and M. Mennuti (1996). Early discharge and home care after unplanned cesarean birth: nursing care time. *Journal of Obstetrics, Gynecology, and Neonatal Nursing* 25(7): 595–600.

This study examined the average nursing time spent planning for early hospital discharge and providing home care to women who delivered by unplanned cesarean birth. It also examined the differences in nursing care time required for patients with and without morbidity when dictated by patient need and provider judgment. Study participants were the treatment group of a larger randomized controlled study ($N = 61$). These were women who had an unplanned cesarean birth, received discharge planning, teaching, and home care follow-up for eight weeks after hospital discharge. In the hospital the nurse specialist evaluated the woman's and newborn's readiness for discharge, coordinated discharge planning, and evaluated the home environment to support recovery and recuperation. After discharge the nurse made at least one home visit during the first week and another during the second week. During the home visits, the nurse performed a physical exam of the mother and infant, evaluated the emotional status, coping, convalescence, parenting, and support systems of the mother. In addition to the home visits, the nurse contacted the family by telephone twice weekly for the first two weeks after discharge, and then weekly for the next six weeks. An advanced practice nurse was available by telephone (8:00 AM to 10:00 PM, Monday through Friday, and 8:00 AM to noon on weekends) for participants to call if they had questions or concerns. All interactions with the mothers, infants, and other family members were recorded in logs maintained for each family. Time was recorded for direct care and indirect care activities. More than half of the women required more than two home visits, with the mean home visit time being one hour. For women who experience morbidity, mean discharge planning time was twenty minutes more, and mean home visit time was forty minutes more than those without morbidity. (No tests of significance were performed.)

This study establishes a link between the amount of time nurses spent caring for patients and nursing care in nonacute care settings. Furthermore, it demonstrated that a method to record nursing time spent on nursing care activities can be applied across treatment settings from hospital to home care to telephone follow-up. The limitations of this study are that it did not have a strong evaluation component of the outcome measure, and no statistical tests were performed to determine significance. This study did not test whether nursing time is a valid or reliable indicator for health care utilization.

Brooten, D., S. Kumar, L.P. Brown, P. Butts, S.A. Finkler, S. Bakewell-Sachs, A. Gibbons, and M. Delivoria-Papadopoulos (1986). A randomized clinical trial of early hospital discharge and home follow-up of very low birthweight infants. *The New England Journal of Medicine* 315(15): 934–9.

(See the section on Strength of Therapeutic Alliance for description of this study.)

The study supported the use of the indicators for family involvement in care planning and decision making and coordination of care processes/continuity of care for the strength of the therapeutic alliance. Additionally, it supported the use of readmission rates as an indicator for utilization. The study was not designed to test the validity or reliability of these indicators, but it did show outcomes for infant care are positively impacted by a nursing intervention which took place in a nonacute care setting. Additionally, with the differences between the treatment and control groups, the study demonstrated that the indicators are responsive.

Brooten, D., M. Naylor, L. Brown, R. York, A. Hollingsworth, S. Cohen, M. Roncoli, and B. Jacobsen (1996). Profile of postdischarge rehospitalizations and acute care visits for seven patient groups. *Public Health Nursing* 13(2): 128–34.

This study examines postdischarge rehospitalization and acute care visits for seven high-risk, high-volume, high-cost patient groups. Participants for the study were taken from treatment groups of other studies that randomized patients into treatment (that is, nurse specialist transitional care) or control (that is, usual care). Participants were categorized into the following patient groups: (1) very low birth weight (n = 79), (2) women with unplanned cesarean birth (n = 122), (3) infants of women who had unplanned cesarean deliveries (n = 123), (4) pregnant women with diabetes (n = 55), (5) women posthysterectomy surgery (n = 109), (6) elderly people with medical cardiac DRGs (n = 142), and (7) people with surgical cardiac DRGs (n = 134). All were drawn from an east coast urban tertiary hospital. As part of each trial, data were collected on the number of rehospitalizations and acute care visits. Acute care visits were defined as emergency room, walk-in, or unscheduled physician visits. Patients in the treatment group received comprehensive discharge planning, a series of home visits, telephone outreach, and daily telephone access to a nurse specialist. Data were collected from the time of discharge to the end of the time for normally expected physical recovery or stabilization for each group. Very low birth weight infants were followed for eighteen months; women who had unplanned cesarean births, their infants, and women who had posthysterectomy surgery were followed for eight weeks; pregnant women with diabetes were followed through their pregnancy; and elderly with medical and surgical DRGs were followed for three months postdischarge. The lowest rate of rehospitalization occurred in the cesarean group (2 percent), while the highest rate occurred in the pregnant women with diabetes (35 percent). (No tests of significance were performed.)

This study shows the relationship between acute and nonacute care nursing activities and rehospitalization rates, emergency room/acute care visit rates, and home visit rates. Because the data used in this study rely on data from other studies (that is, a secondary analysis), the article does not explain the methodology for obtaining and calculating rehospitalization, acute care visit rate, and home visit information. In addition, this study did not test the validity or reliability of this information in measuring health care utilization.

H. Kitzman, D. L. Olds, C. R. Henderson, C. Hanks, R. Cole, R. Tatelbaum, K. M. McConnochie, K. Sidora, D. W. Luckey, W. Shaver, K. Engelhardt, D. James, and K. Barnard (1997). Effect of prenatal and infancy home visitation by nurses on pregnancy outcomes, childhood injuries, and repeated childbearing. *Journal of the American Medical Association* 278(8): 644–53.

This study tested the effect of prenatal and infancy home visits by nurses on pregnancy-induced hypertension, preterm delivery, low birth weight, children's injuries, immunizations, mental development, behavioral problems, and maternal life courses. This was a randomized controlled trial conducted in the public system of obstetric care in Memphis, Tennessee. From June 1, 1990 to August 31, 1991, 1,290 consecutive women from the obstetrical clinic at the Regional Medical Center in Memphis were invited to the study. The women were less than twenty-nine weeks pregnant and had no previous live births, no specific chronic illnesses thought to contribute to fetal growth retardation or preterm delivery, and at least two of several identified socioeconomic risk factors. Sample size was set from a series of power calculations in which alpha = .05 and beta = .20 and two-tailed tests were specified. Subjects included 1,139 primarily African-American women at less than 29 weeks' gestation with no previous live births and at least two sociodemographic risk characteristics. The women were divided into four treatment groups. The first group received prenatal care but no postpartum visits. The second treatment group received prenatal care and developmental screening and services for the child at 6, 12, and 24 months of age. The third group was provided intensive nursing home visitation services during pregnancy, three screening visits, one postpartum visit in the hospital before discharge, and one postpartum visit at home. The final group of women received the same services as the women in the third group and continued to receive home visits through the child's second birthday. For the individuals in the fourth treatment group, nurses made an average of seven home visits during pregnancy and twenty-six more visits between the date of delivery and the child's second birthday. Data were collected by interviews with the mothers and abstractions of medical and social services records. The individuals collecting the data were unaware of the women's treatment group assignments. Medical records were abstracted to capture information about pregnancy-induced hypertension, preterm delivery, low birth weight, children's injuries, ingestions, and immunizations. The subjects were interviewed at the time of registration, the 28th and 36th weeks of pregnancy, and at the children's 6th, 12th, and 24th months of life to gather information about the children's behavioral problems and the mother's subsequent pregnancies, educational achievement, and workforce participation. Use of welfare services was derived from state records, and the children's mental health was tested at the 24th-month office visit using the Bayley scales of infant development, and their mothers completed the Achenbach Child Behavior Checklist. The major findings of the study were that the women in the fourth treatment group had lower rates of pregnancy-induced hypertension (13 percent versus 20 percent; $p = .009$);

healthcare encounters for children in which injuries or ingestions were detected (.43 versus .55; $p = .05$); days that the children were hospitalized with injuries or ingestions (.03 versus .16; $p < .001$); and second pregnancies (36 percent versus 47 percent; $p = .006$). There were no significant program effects on any of the other variables tested.

This study demonstrated that home nursing visits can lead to decreased healthcare use by reducing both the number of emergency room visits and hospital admission rates. The study also demonstrated that the availability of prenatal and postpartum home nursing care can lead to an increase in protective factors, resulting in a decrease in injuries to the child. The differences in the results achieved by the different treatment groups demonstrates the validity, sensitivity, and responsiveness of the number and appropriateness of emergency room visits, hospital admission rates, and a decrease in injuries as indicators of the quality or availability of nursing care.

Martens, K.H., and S.D. Mellor (1997). A study of the relationship between home care services and hospital readmissions of patients with congestive heart failure. *Home Healthcare Nurse* 15(2): 123–9.

This study examined the relationship between home care nursing services and hospital readmissions for patients admitted with a primary diagnosis of congestive heart failure (CHF). The study was retrospective, exploratory, and descriptive and used a computerized database of medical records database obtained from two hospitals in Columbus, Ohio. A sample of 924 discharges from the hospitals to the home were identified for the one-year period June 1, 1993 to May 31, 1994. About a quarter of the sample (26.7 percent) was referred to a home care agency. This group received an average of 10.74 visits by a registered nurse during the ninety-day period after discharge with CHF from the hospital. A total of 161 patients were readmitted between one and six times within ninety days of discharge. A chi-square analysis showed that patients receiving home care services were readmitted to the hospital less often within a ninety-day period after discharge than those patients not receiving home care services. The shorter the period after discharge, however, the less significant the difference in readmission rates between the home care and non–home care group.

The results and the literature presented in this study demonstrate that home health nursing services is a strong predictor for hospital readmissions, thereby demonstrating a link between nonacute care nursing care and hospital readmissions. In addition, it supports the responsive and generalizability of readmission rates as an indicator for health service utilization. Limitations of the study are that it did not use a randomized controlled trial methodology, so there may be event biases that contribute to the significant results that were reported, and a lack of information exists about any differences in the severity of illness or the cost of services. This study did not test the reliability or sensitivity of the indicator to health service utilization.

Miller, L.L., M.C. Hornbrook, P.G. Archbold, and B.J. Stewart (1996). Development of use and cost measures in a nursing intervention for family caregivers and frail elderly patients. *Research in Nursing and Health* 19: 273–85.

This study compared the cost and utilization of a home health nursing intervention called PREP to usual home health nursing care. PREP nursing care differed from standard home health nursing care in that it focused on the caregiver/care receiver dyad, addressed all health problems experienced by the dyad, focused on increasing predictability in caregiving processes, and provided follow-up and monitoring over an extended time period. The sample included eleven dyads randomized into the intervention (PREP) and control (usual care) groups. At baseline, the intervention and control groups differed significantly in that the control care receivers were younger (mean age 74 versus 80) and control caregivers were younger (mean age 62 versus 73.5) than their corresponding intervention group. A comprehensive service utilization profile and associated costs were calculated for each dyad. The utilization profile contained thirty-eight services for care receivers and six services for caregivers, including PREP nursing services, standard home-health services (physical, occupational, and speech therapy as well as social work, home health aid, homemaker), institutional services (hospital, nursing home, adult foster home), emergency services, ambulance, outpatient services, community social services, pharmacy, durable medical equipment, and medical supplies. Utilization and cost data were collected from three sources: (1) HMO computer files, (2) member outpatient records, and (3) study participants. HMO computer files contained most of the institutional services and outpatient services. Medical outpatient records were used to identify telephone calls to advise nurses (non-PREP, HMO nurses). Study participants provided information monthly for the duration of the project on out-of-pocket expenses, expenses for non-HMO services for caregivers who were not members of the HMO, and services received from community social services. The duration of the project ranged from three to six months for the dyads in the sample. Presumably, because of the small sample size used in this study, service use was not expressed in terms of rate but in absolute numbers (such as number of visits, admissions, days). As anticipated, the PREP program participants had fewer hospital days, ALOS for hospital stay, long-term care days and lower rates of ambulance and pharmacy use as well as lower associated costs. However, none of the results were statistically significant (t-tests with one-tailed p-value).

This study showed a trend in favor of the PREP program as measured by favorable utilization patterns and decreased costs. It showed how a non-acute care nursing intervention may impact service use and identifies the types of service use that would be effected. It also demonstrates how utilization of various services, as they are defined in this article, differs by treatment and control groups, which indicates that these utilization measures may be responsive to change in the intervention. The finding of statistically insignificant differences between intervention and control may be explained by the small sample size or the age differences between the groups. The methods of data collection, specifically relying on patient participation, may be more difficult and costly in studies with larger sample sizes.

Olds, D., C.R. Henderson, H. Kitzman, and R. Cole (1995). Effects of prenatal and infancy nursing home visitation on surveillance of child maltreatment. *Pediatrics* 95(3): 365–72.

This study examined the long-term effects of a prenatal and infancy nursing home visitation program on child abuse and neglect. This randomized, controlled trial was conducted in a semirural community in upstate New York. Families located to fourteen other states during the two-year period after the children's second birthdays. The participants included 400 primiparous women entered into the study before their 30th week of pregnancy. The participants were stratified into four different treatment groups. The first group received screening and referral services from an infant specialist. The second group received free transportation for regular prenatal and well-child care at local clinics and physicians' offices as well as the screening and referral services provided to the first group. The individuals in the third group were provided a nurse home visitor during pregnancy in addition to the screening and transportation services. The nurses visited these families approximately every two weeks and made an average of nine visits to each pregnant woman. The average visit lasted one hour and fifteen minutes. The women in the fourth treatment group received the same treatment as the women in the third group and continued home nursing visits until the child's second birthday. The nursing visitation program was designed to improve three aspects of maternal and child functioning: pregnancy outcomes, qualities of parental caregiving, and maternal life-course development. The data were collected by interviewing the women and using the following assessment tools: the Caldwell and Bradley Home Inventory, an observation checklist of the child's exposure to hazards, the Stanford-Binet Form L-M test of intelligence, and a review of Child Protective Service records for New York state and the other fourteen states to which participants relocated. The interviews and assessments were conducted at registration and at the 34th, 36th, 46th, and 48th months of the children's lives. Regression analyses were performed. Estimates and tests were adjusted for all covariates, classification factors, and interactions. This study focused on the fifty-six families in the original group of 400 in which the children had a state-verified report of child abuse or child neglect during the first 4 years of life. There were no statistically significant differences between the families' sociodemographic or psychosocial characteristics before assignment to treatment groups. The nurse-visited maltreated children made 84 percent fewer visits to the physician for injuries ($p = .01$) and ingestions, 38 percent fewer visits to the emergency room ($p = .008$), and their homes were observed to have fewer health hazards ($p = .03$) and to be more educationally and socially stimulating ($p = .07$) than the children in the other treatment groups. In addition, the mothers of the children in the nurse-visited treatment group were less controlling of their children ($p = .02$) and less likely to report that their children used car seats ($p = .03$) and safety belts ($p = .002$) regularly than the women in the comparison groups. In addition, the nurse-visited cases had fewer indications of "lack of supervision" in the maltreatment record than did the other cases ($p = .03$). Three of the four identified cases of sexual abuse occurred among nurse-visited families.

This study demonstrated that home nursing visits can lead to decreased healthcare utilization by reducing both the number of emergency room visits and hospital admission rates. The study also demonstrated that the availability of prenatal and postpartum home nursing care can lead to an increase in protective factors, resulting in a decrease in injuries to the child. The differences in the results achieved by the different treatment groups demonstrates the validity, sensitivity, and responsiveness of the number and appropriateness of emergency room visits and hospital admission rates, and a decrease in injuries as indicators of the quality or availability of nursing care.

Weinberger, M., E.Z. Oddone, and W.G. Henderson (1996). Does increased access to primary care reduce hospital readmissions? *The New England Journal of Medicine* 334(22): 1441–7.

This study measured rehospitalization, quality of life, and satisfaction with care after implementing an intensive primary care delivery model on patients admitted to a general medicine service unit at one of the nine Veteran's Affairs (VA) medical centers. Of the patients admitted for diabetes, chronic obstructive pulmonary disease, or congestive heart failure, 1,396 patients were randomly assigned to treatment (primary care intervention) or control (usual care) groups. The intervention involved close follow-up by a nurse and a primary care physician beginning at some point before discharge and continuing for the next 6 months after discharge. The samples were stratified by entitlement status (which can affect access to primary care) and disease. The authors report no significant differences between treatment ($n = 695$) and control ($n = 701$) groups with respect to age, education level, marital status, race, gender, employment status, length of index admission, time from randomization to discharge, eligibility status, hospital days in the 180 days prior to the index admission, index diagnosis, disease status, or risk for readmission (based on validated measure of coexisting conditions). Utilization of VA services within 180 days after discharge from the index hospitalization was assessed by reviewing computerized hospitalization and outpatient visit files. Satisfaction with care (using 11 scales from a patient satisfaction questionnaire) and quality of life (using the short form of the SF-36) was assessed during a phone call to the patient 30 days and 180 days after randomization. Contrary to the study's hypothesis, the results showed that the treatment group actually had significantly *higher* readmission rates (0.19 versus 0.14 per month; $p = .005$, using Wilcoxon rank-sum tests) and days of rehospitalization (10.2 versus 8.8; $p = .041$, using Wilcoxon rank-sum test) than the control group. However, patients in the treatment group were more satisfied with their care ($p < .001$, using multivariate analysis of covariance), but there was no significant difference between the two groups in terms of their quality of life, which remained very low throughout the study. The authors added that while the treatment group made more visits to general medicine clinics ($p < .001$), it also made significantly fewer visits to subspecialty clinics ($p = .01$). In terms of the intensity of the primary care intervention, the mean number of days between discharge after the index hospitalization and the first visit to a general medicine clinic was significantly shorter for the intervention group ($p < .001$), and the treatment group was more likely to visit at least one general medicine clinic during the study period ($p < .001$). Primary care nurses talked with patients in the treatment group by telephone a mean of 7.5 times during the study period, for an average of 5.7 minutes per call.

The intervention, involving nursing and medicine in both acute and nonacute care setting, and the outcome measures (readmission, outpatient visits, nursing time) demonstrate the link between these outcome measures and the quality of nursing care in nonacute care settings. The limitations of this study are that it did not test the validity and reliability of these outcome measures to the area of health service utilization. The differences between the treatment and control groups, however, demonstrate that these measures are responsive and likely to be generalizable.

5. Client/Patient Satisfaction

Baradell, J.G. (1995). Clinical outcomes and satisfaction of patients of clinical nurse specialists in psychiatric-mental health nursing. *Archives of Psychiatric Nursing* IX(5): 240–50.

The results of this study demonstrated the relationship between symptom management/relief cognition, psychological/neurological/cognitive functioning, communication, satisfaction with social functioning, satisfaction with role functioning, satisfaction with family coping, and satisfaction with quality of care rendered and the quality or availability of nursing care. (See the section on Changes in Symptom Severity for a description of this study.)

Graveley, E.A., and J.H. Littlefield (1992). A cost-effectiveness analysis of three staffing models for the delivery of low-risk prenatal care. *American Journal of Public Health* 82(2): 180–4.

This study performed a comparative cost-effectiveness analysis of three low-risk prenatal clinic staffing models: (1) physician-based (MDC), (2) mixed staffing, including a physician, nurse practitioner, registered nurses, and nurses aids (MSC), and (3) nurse-based (RNC). Three separate clinics were identified for each of the staffing models and 52 subjects from each clinic were included in the study. The total sample size ($N = 156$) was determined from a power analysis of 3 months of birth-weight data from women who attended the clinics and delivered at the county hospital. The sample was drawn over a 3-month period in 1989 from women who delivered at the county hospital. To be included in the study, the participants had to be 18 years or older; obtain their prenatal care at one of the clinics, with a minimum of 3 prenatal visits; and deliver within 48 hours of the interview. Four broad-based categories of patient variables were analyzed, including demographics, physiological measures, satisfaction with care, and cost. The authors chose to use the patient satisfaction tool (PST) to assess maternal satisfaction with access to care. This is a 27-item survey that uses a 6-point Likert scale and addressed 5 areas of satisfaction with care: accessibility, affordability, availability, acceptability, and accommodations. In other studies, the internal consistency reliability coefficient was reported as .83. Subjects from the RNC clinic were significantly less likely to be Hispanic, more likely to have graduated from high school, and more likely to be on Medicaid than subjects in the other two clinics. Analysis of variance (ANOVA) was performed to assess the relationship between these demographic variables and patient satisfaction, and no significant relationships were found for Medicaid coverage and ethnicity. However, educational level was statistically significant for two of the PST statements, including the statements, "I saw the same physician/registered nurse for all my prenatal care," and "the fees at the clinic were more than I wanted to pay." The PST internal reliability coefficient in this study was .76, and ANOVA tests revealed no significant differences among the clinics for the satisfaction areas of accessibility and affordability. However, a Student Newman-Keuls post hoc *t*-test showed significant differences among the clinics for the other areas of satisfaction. In general, the RNC was found to have greater scores for satisfaction with availability, acceptability, accommodation, and total satisfaction. The RNC had significantly higher scores (no *p*-values reported) for accommodation and total satisfaction as compared to the MDC. And the RNC had significantly higher scores on all measures compared to the MSC.

The results of this study support the link between the availability of nursing care and patient satisfaction with the accessibility, communication, and skill mix. This study supported the reliability, generalizability, and responsiveness of the PST tool. In addition, there is a link between the scales of the PST tool and nonacute care nursing.

Jacox, A.K., B.R. Bausell, and D.M. Mahrenholz (1997). Patient satisfaction with nursing care in hospitals. *Outcomes Management in Nursing Practice.* 1(1):20–8.

The study was based on the premise that measures of patient satisfaction with nursing care needed to more clearly distinguish among dimensions of patient satisfaction with nursing care. The dimensions studied were based on those originally studied by Risser (1975), and included caring, technical skill, and patient education. This article reported on two pilot studies and one major study. In the first pilot study, 200 patients were identified from a list of discharged patients from 9 medical-surgical units at a mid-Atlantic teaching hospital. Patients were randomly assigned into those completing the form before leaving the hospital and those completing the form after leaving the hospital (Those patients mailed the forms back in stamped, addressed envelopes). There was an overall 70 percent response rate, with a higher response rate from those who completed the form before leaving the hospital. The ratings were markedly skewed toward the positive end, with 75 percent of the responses being 5 (completely satisfied). Using five-item scales for the three dimensions of care, the authors found that the internal consistency reliabilities were .95, .91, and .94, respectively, for the caring, technical, and teaching domains. No significant differences were identified between any of the demographic variables and the scales; additionally, no significant differences were identified between the two data collection modalities, although the in-hospital ratings tended to be higher. To validate these findings, a second pilot study was conducted in another hospital in the same city. In this pilot, four different instruments were used: five-point scale with instructions to "not mark all 5's or all 1's"; five-point scale with no such instructions; seven-point scale with complete instructions based on the number of responses; and a seven-point scale without the special instruction. Two hundred subjects were randomly assigned to receive one of the four instruments. No significant differences were identified between the two types of instruction or the two types of scales with respect to skewness. Internal consistency was high again for the scales (numbers not given). In the major study, 2,892 patients were asked to complete a revised 19-item survey. Selection criteria included: 1 of 12 targeted, high-volume diagnosis-related groupings; discharged alive from 1 of 5 Midwestern hospitals; and complete nursing care data had been collected on them during their hospitalization. The effective response rate was 50.2 percent (method of collection is not mentioned). The results indicated that caring, nursing skill, and patient education are three distinct dimensions of nursing care. A weak positive relationship was found for age ($r = .07$; $p < .01$), indicating that older people tended to give higher ratings in their satisfaction with nursing care. The authors also examined correlations with overall hospital satisfaction and differences between units and hospitals.

This study supports the validity, reliability, and generalizability of measures of patient satisfaction with quality of nursing care rendered. There is a direct link to nursing care, but the studies were conducted in acute care settings and it is unclear whether the results would be substantiated if similar studies were conducted in nonacute care settings. There was no use of control groups in which to measure the responsiveness of the indicator.

Ketefian, S., R. Redman, M.G. Nash, and E.L. Bogue (1997). Inpatient and ambulatory patient satisfaction with nursing care. *Quality Management in Health Care* 5(4): 66–75.

This study reported the development and psychometric testing of an inpatient and ambulatory patient satisfaction survey. The surveys measured patient satisfaction using standards of nursing practice within the University of Michigan Medical Center. The dimensions of nursing care that were tested in the survey included preprocedure information, nursing care, management of pain and discomfort, discharge planning and process, planning and teaching for care at home, and courteous treatment of family (inpatient). The inpatient survey contained 32 items, and the ambulatory survey contained 33 items. Each item required a response on a Likert-type scale of 1 (strongly agree) to 5 (strongly disagree). Surveys were administered 4 to 6 weeks after discharge from the hospital or after a clinic visit so that all aspects of care could be evaluated. Two waves of survey data-gathering occurred from all units, with sample sizes from each proportional to the volume of patients on the unit. In total, there were 619 inpatient and 955 ambulatory surveys completed (out of 1,561 and 2,970 surveys mailed, respectively). Factor analyses suggested the existence of four scales for inpatient and five scales for outpatient satisfaction with high reliability and reasonable validity. The five scales of outpatient satisfaction included general satisfaction with nursing care, general dissatisfaction with nursing care, management of pain and discomfort, information on procedures and follow-up care, and emergency room communication and care. Cronbach's alphas ranged from .84 to .96 for the ambulatory scales. Construct correlation and intercorrelations were also moderate to high.

This survey demonstrated the validity and reliability of a patient satisfaction survey used to measure patient satisfaction with the quality of nursing care rendered and satisfaction with communication with caregivers. There was a clear link to nursing in that this survey was specifically designed to assess satisfaction with nursing care, and a clear link was established to nursing care in nonacute care settings. The results were skewed toward favorable responses, but the authors created a dichotomous variable to correct the skewed results. Sensitivity or responsiveness of the surveys cannot be ascertained from this article.

Lowry, L., J. Saeger, and S. Barnett (1997). Client Satisfaction with prenatal care and pregnancy outcomes. *Outcomes Management for Nursing Practice* 1(1): 29–35.

This study determined whether nursing case management improved pregnancy outcomes and client satisfaction for pregnant women of low socioeconomic status. Two initiatives were implemented in the state of Florida. One was an Improved Pregnancy Outcome Program (IPOP) delivered through the Human Resource Service County Public Health Clinics, and the other was a multidisciplinary ambulatory healthcare center for women and children (MDC). The IPOP clinic used advanced practice nurses (APNs) to deliver care in conjunction with an attending obstetrician on call fore obstetric or medical problems. The MDC utilized case management Registered Nurses (RNs) and APNs to serve as case managers for clients who received care from a team made up of RNs, APNs, obstetricians, gynecologists, social workers, nutrition counselors, and health educators. The first 62 pregnant clients from each clinic who were English-speaking, literate, and had given voluntary consent were invited to participate in the study during the fall of 1994. Clients with three or more clinic visits were asked to complete the Risser Patient Satisfaction Scale, developed to measure patient attitudes toward nurses and nursing care in ambulatory clinic settings. A new subscale of six items measuring factors related to setting was added to the Raiser instrument for the purposes of this study. The new subscale and the other three Risser scales were pilot tested on 30 of the pregnant clients, 15 from each clinic. Alpha coefficients for the pre- and post-tests were .79 and .74 , respectively. Test–retest reliability was calculated, yielding an overall Pearson correlation coefficient of .86. Independent sample *t*-tests of means calculated for technical skill, teaching, interpersonal relationships, and setting indicated significant differences between treatment settings. Clients from the MDC group were more likely to agree with positive statements about nurses' technical skill teaching, and interpersonal relationships than were those from the PHC. There were no significant differences in healthcare outcomes between the two groups.

This study demonstrated the sensitivity, reliability, and responsiveness of satisfaction with quality of care rendered, and satisfaction with communication as indicators of satisfaction with quality of care. In addition, the study established a link between the quality or availability of nursing care in an outpatient setting and patient satisfaction.

Ludwig-Behmer, P., C.J. Ryan, N.J. Johnson, K.A. Hennessy, M.C. Gattuso, R. Epsom, and K.T. Czurylo. (1993). Using patient perceptions to improve quality care. *Journal of Nursing Care Quality* 7(2): 42–51.

This study defined patient perceptions of quality care and caring and compared patient satisfaction with quality of care using three methods of data collection: unsolicited letters, patient satisfaction questionnaire, and general quality of care survey. The satisfaction questionnaire was designed by a nursing quality improvement and research committee at a medical center in Illinois (the questionnaire was included in the article). Content validity was established by a review panel of experts. It was pilot tested, but no attempts were made to formally establish reliability. The questionnaire was administered at the time of discharge to a convenience sample of patients ($N = 444$). The questionnaire contained five questions with four-item responses ranging from *never* to *always*; two questions with four-item responses from *poor* to *excellent*; two behavioral-intention questions with yes/no responses; and two open-ended questions. Most of the questions were general to nursing care, including attentiveness of nursing staff; length of time to respond to requests; knowledge of nurses; explanations about medications, procedures, and routines; courteousness of nursing staff; and overall rating of nursing care. The authors only reported on two of the patient satisfaction questionnaire items, demonstrating how the responses obtained from the questionnaire were similar to the responses obtained from the quality of care survey. No description of the quality of care survey is provided, nor is there information about the population to which the survey was administered. The authors stated that it was developed by another group (Carey and Posavac 1982) and construct validity, predictive validity, and reliability have been established.

The validity of a patient satisfaction tool to measure satisfaction with nursing care quality, communication, and staff mix was supported in this article. Although the questionnaire was administered to patients in an acute care setting, the questions on the survey may be applicable to patients in the nonacute care settings as well. Additional, more rigorous testing of the survey tool would be necessary to demonstrate its reliability, responsiveness, and generalizability.

Paykel, E.S., S.P. Mangen, J.H. Griffith, and T.P. Burns (1982). Community psychiatric nursing for neurotic patients: a controlled trial. *British Journal of Psychiatry* 140: 573–81.

This study determined whether there was a difference in outcomes for patients receiving routine outpatient psychiatric care as opposed to those receiving home visits by psychiatric nurses. The nursing was based at Springfield Hospital, London, a psychiatric hospital serving a local catchment area of 350,000. Outpatient clinics were held at several large hospital clinics and two smaller clinics in the London area. Eight full-time, psychiatric nurses were involved in the study. They worked in coordination with 10 catchment area teams, and in most cases they worked exclusively with one team. The sample consisted of patients being discharged from the hospital or having already completed 6 months of outpatient treatment. All subjects had

International Classification of Diseases, ninth edition (ICD-9) diagnoses of neuroses, unipolar affective psychoses, or anankastic, hysterical, or asthenic personality disorders. All subjects were determined by the treatment team to be in need of at least 6 months of further follow-up care. All outpatient clinic attendees and impending hospital/day hospital discharges were screened for inclusion in the study. After initial assessment, suitable subjects were randomly assigned to one of the two treatment groups using a minimization procedure, which allowed matching on 14 demographic, diagnostic, history, and current rating variables. Treatment was continued for up to 18 months, and subjects who completed less than 6 months of treatment were dropped from the study. Contacts with the nurse and the precise nature of those contacts were as clinically indicated. Assessments were conducted by the research sociologist and psychologist not involved in the treatment. These took place initially and at 6-month intervals until the 18th month. Symptom assessments were made using the Clinical Interview for Depression, the Raskin Three Area Depression Scale, and the Covi Three Area Anxiety Scale. Social adjustment was assessed using the Social Adjustment Scale. Satisfaction was assessed at each interview with the patient and relative on a number of specific and global aspects. In addition, at the end of 18 months, the client completed a self-report questionnaire for consumer satisfaction. A reliability study between the two raters, on the interview symptom ratings and the Social Adjustment Scale, showed mean correlations of .82 and .85, respectively. A total of 99 patients were included in the main study sample. Seventy-one patients completed a full 18 months, with 36 in community psychiatric nursing and 35 in outpatient care. No differences were found in the effectiveness of the two modes of treatment on symptoms, social adjustment, or family burden. Community psychiatric resulted in a reduction in outpatient contacts with psychiatrists and other staff, a slight increase in contacts with general practitioners for prescriptions, and an improvement in patient satisfaction. A total of 46 percent of the group receiving community psychiatric care and 72 percent of the group receiving routine outpatient care was still receiving psychiatric care at the conclusion of 18 months of treatment. While the differences in overall patient satisfaction were not statistically significant, there was a statistically significant difference in the patients' satisfaction with the quality of care received $< .05$ and communication $< .05$, with the patients receiving psychiatric nursing care being more satisfied than those receiving routine outpatient care.

This study supported the validity, reliability, sensitivity, and responsiveness of patient satisfaction with quality of care rendered and patient satisfaction with communication as indicators of patient satisfaction. In addition, this study established a link between the quality or availability of nursing care in a community care setting and patient satisfaction with communication and patient satisfaction with quality of care rendered. The limitations of this study included the small sample size, the lack of information about potential confounding factors, and the lack of detailed information about the content of the patient satisfaction tools.

Rhee, K.J., and A.L. Dermyer (1995). Patient satisfaction with a nurse practitioner in a university emergency service. *Annals of Emergency Medicine* 26(2): 130–2.

This study measured overall satisfaction of patients who saw a nurse practitioner (NP) compared to patients who were seen in the usual fashion at an emergency department (ED) in a large urban medical center. A telephone survey of patients who were seen by the NP over a two-month period was conducted to assess overall satisfaction, satisfaction with technical and humanistic aspects of physician and nursing care, impression of the cleanliness of the ED, convenience of parking, and other aspects of ED service. Phone calls were made within 2 months of the ED visit by a single investigator. Forty percent of patients (or parents in the case of children and incompetent adults) was not available or unreachable by telephone. For each of the 30 patients that were seen by an NP and reached by telephone, a control patient was identified, matching by date, time of service, intensity of service (per billing code), and person responding (that is, patient or parent). The groups were not significantly different in age or sex. A five-point scale ranging from excellent (5) to poor (1) developed by Ware (see Ware article) was used to quantify overall patient satisfaction. Overall satisfaction was good for both groups and not significantly different (3.9 for the NP group and 4.0 for the control group; $p = .66$ using contingency-table analysis). These results suggests that patients were equally satisfied being seen by an NP or physician in the emergency department.

This article showed how satisfaction with communication, access, quality, and skill mix can be linked to nursing services, and that these are responsive and generalizable measures. However, it did not test whether these indicators are valid or reliable ways to measure overall patient satisfaction.

Safran, D.G., A.R. Tarlov, and W. H. Rogers (1994). Primary care performance in fee-for-service and prepaid health care systems: results from the medical outcomes study. *The Journal of the American Medical Association.* 271(20): 1579–86.

In this study, the authors examined the differences in the quality of primary care delivered in prepaid, health maintenance organizations (HMOs) independent practice associations (IPA), and fee-for service (FFS) health care systems. In particular, there were seven components of satisfaction investigated, building from five core dimensions of high-quality care defined by the Institute of Medicine. The seven components in this study were accessibility (financial and organizational), continuity, comprehensiveness, coordination, and accountability (interpersonal and technical). The accessibility and accountability scales were demonstrated to be valid in other research. The validity of the other scales in previous research was not discussed. Subjects were identified from a longitudinal panel of the Medical Outcomes Study (MOS), which was conducted in three large cities between 1986 and 1990 using a variety of adult patients who received care from a family medicine, general internal medicine, endocrinology, cardiology, or psychiatry physician; nurse practitioner; or social worker. The patients were included in the panel if they had one of five clinical tracer conditions: hypertension, diabetes, congestive heart failure, recent myocardial infarction, or major depressive disorder. They were excluded from the study sample if they had only a mental illness tracer condition with no physical tracer condition; their MOS provider was not their primary care provider; or data on health care payment system were not available. Nearly half of the study sample ($N = 1{,}208$) were from FFS systems ($n = 625$); a third ($n = 463$) were from HMO systems; and the remaining were from IPA systems ($n = 120$). On average, FFS patients were older and sicker than HMO and IPA patients. HMO patients were less likely to receive primary care from a medical specialist and more likely to have a female primary care physician than patients in FFS or IPA systems. These differences were controlled for by the regression analysis of patient satisfaction. The regression showed that patients with prepaid care (HMO or IPA) were more satisfied with their financial access than patients with FFS care ($p < .001$). Organizational access, continuity, and accountability were highest in FFS systems ($p < .05$, and coordination was highest ($p < .05$) and comprehensiveness was lowest ($p < .001$) in patients in HMO systems.

This study demonstrated that these measures of patient satisfaction with access were valid indicators for patient satisfaction. The differences observed in the different payment systems demonstrated that the indicators were responsive. There was a clear link to satisfaction measures in non acute care settings, as satisfaction with primary care was assessed in this study. A link to nursing, however, was less strongly supported by this study in that satisfaction with care was assessed for physicians, nurses, or social workers but there is no indication how many nurses were included in the study. The variety of patients seen in this study supported generalizability, but reliability and sensitivity were not specifically addressed.

Ross, C.K., C.A. Steward, and J.M. Sinacore (1995). A comparative study of seven measures of patient satisfaction. *Medical Care* 33(4): 392–406.

This study examined the extent to which seven commonly used measures of satisfaction agreed in levels of satisfaction obtained. The subjects included in the study were randomly selected from patients scheduled for an outpatient visit at a large urban Veterans Administration (VA) hospital. Patients were pulled from medical (general and subspecialty), surgical, dental, and nonphysician managed clinics at the VA hospital. A total of 233 patients was interviewed (84 percent response rate) on 7 different measures of patient satisfaction. The seven measures were single-item evaluation of overall quality (global rating); a 29-item multidimensional evaluation of quality, including access, availability, technical quality of care, interpersonal care, communication, and financial; a 2-item overall evaluation of quality of care; 10 items that measure attitude of general satisfaction and satisfaction with physician; 4 measures of behavioral intention, including willingness to return for care, refer to a friend, report that the quality of care was excellent, and follow the doctors' recommendations; 2 willingness-to-pay questions; and measures of acquiescent response bias. In addition, during the interview a 138-item sickness impact profile was conducted to assess functional status. The patients sampled ranged in age from 21 to 87 years, with a mean age of 61.5, were predominantly male (97 percent), and nearly half (43 percent) did not complete high school.

The study found that the best measures of patient satisfaction were the global rating, the multidimensional evaluation of quality, and the overall satisfaction. In addition, this study supports the validity and reliability of access to care as an indicator of patient satisfaction. However, the authors note that there is substantial variation in the conclusions about the patients' satisfaction related to specific types of measures used and the difficulty of response bias. In addition, this study was not linked to nursing care.

Ware, J.E., and R.D. Hays (1988). Method for measuring patient satisfaction with specific medical encounters. *Medical Care* 26(4): 393–402.

In this article, two corresponding studies are reported by the authors. In one study, the authors compared a commonly used method with an infrequently used method for measuring patient satisfaction with a specific medical encounter. A group of 136 patient volunteers from outpatient visiting fee-for-service clinics were asked to complete a 51-item booklet containing the visit-specific satisfaction questionnaire (VSQ). The average age of the group was 41.8 years and 75 percent were female. The median annual income was $6,000; 13 percent reported incomes over $30,000. About four out of five patients had used the clinic before; most reported seeing their doctor regularly. Item response format was manipulated so that some respondents were administered a six-item response scale (that is, S6, which included *extremely satisfied*, *very satisfied*, *somewhat satisfied*, *neither satisfied nor dissatisfied*, *somewhat dissatisfied*, and *very dissatisfied*), and some were administered a five-item scale (that is, E5, which *included excellent*, *very good*, *good*, *fair*, and *poor*). Both the E5 and S6 measures assessed satisfaction with the visit overall; the technical quality (thoroughness, carefulness, competency) of the doctor and completeness of service; the interpersonal manner (courtesy, respect, sensitivity, friendliness) of the doctor and; the length of time waiting in the office for the visit. Additionally, the location of the satisfaction questions (that is, the VSQ portion of the survey) was manipulated to determine if greater satisfaction was reported when satisfaction questions included demographic and descriptive questions as well as questions about the visit. Finally, each questionnaire contained four measures used to test validity: continuity of care; how the visit compared with previous visits; three behavioral intentions; and three items measuring general satisfaction, technical care, and interpersonal care selected from the Patient Satisfaction Questionnaire. Questionnaires with different response scales and location of VSQ were randomly distributed to the participants. The mean scores for the E5 scale were significantly lower than the S6 format for ratings of office wait time. The same trend was observed for the other measures of care, but these differences were not statistically significant.

Both response scales yielded satisfactory estimates of internal consistency reliability. Correlations between the E5 and S6 response scale ratings for each of the four main areas of satisfaction and the eight items selected for measuring validity showed that most (62 of 64 correlations) were in the hypothesized direction, supporting the validity of both rating methods. However, the E5 measures generally showed stronger correlations than did the S6 measures to the validity variables. Finally, in this first study, the authors found that, indeed, having the patients respond to demographic and descriptive questions about their visit before rating their satisfaction yielded less favorable satisfaction scores. In the second study, the questionnaire (with the addition of a few more validity variables) was administered to patients in other clinical settings (that is, Internal Medicine, Medical Specialties, and Surgical Specialties in an HMO on the East Coast). Again, internal consistency was high for both the E5 and S6 response formats, and the E5 generally outperformed the S6 when measuring the four areas of patient satisfaction.

This study demonstrated the validity of both the E5 and S6 formats for questions related to satisfaction with care management/treatment regimen, satisfaction with transition across treatment settings, satisfaction with the quality of care rendered, and satisfaction with access to care in that they were correlated with other measures of satisfaction. It also demonstrated the reliability and generalizability of these indicators. However, it did not test the responsiveness or sensitivity of these indicators.

6. Risk Reduction (Environmental and Behavioral)

Anderson, B., J. Ho, J. Brackett, D. Finkelstein, and L. Laffel (1997). Parental involvement in diabetes management tasks: relationships to blood glucose monitoring adherence and metabolic control in young adolescents with insulin-dependent diabetes mellitus. *The Journal of Pediatrics* 130(2): 257–65.

The direct link between nursing care and patient compliance with treatment plans and involvement of caregivers is not explicitly stated, but general patient compliance to treatment regimens and self-care are considered areas of nursing practice. The context of the intervention, targeting caregiver involvement, and the results of the study (that is, better glycemic control) support the validity of the involvement of a primary care giver as an indicator of increased protective factors and the involvement of a primary caregiver as an indicator of risk reduction. The reliability of these was demonstrated by the fact that there was a 94 percent inter-rater reliability. The involvement also showed responsiveness: the children of less involved parents (older age group) had higher total glycosolated hemoglobin counts. It is unclear from this article, but it may be assumed that these findings are sensitive and generalizable. (See the section on Increase in Protective Factors for the description of this study.)

Barry, K. (1993). Patient self-medication: an innovative approach to medication teaching. *Journal of Nursing Care Quality* 8(1): 75–82.

This study developed, implemented, and evaluated a self-medication program that would increase patients' knowledge of medication, participation in care, and compliance with their medication regimen after discharge from a general surgical and transplantation unit. A four-phase program was developed and an assessment tool was administered pre- and post-test implementation to determine if there were changes in patients' knowledge of their medication regimens. In the first phase of the program, the patients' verbal consent was obtained, medications were reviewed, and physician order to participate in the study was obtained. In the second phase, the nurse and patient developed a mutually agreeable medication schedule in accordance with the physician's recommendations. Verbal and written information about medications was provided. In the third phase, the pharmacist provided medication labels. The nurse placed the labels on plastic bags with the appropriate medications for a 24-hour period, and then gave the bags to the patient. The patient took the medication independently, and the nurse performed a pill count every eight hours to see that the patient was taking medications appropriately. The final phase of the program involved the nurse administering the assessment tool of patients' knowledge of their medication regimen at the time of discharge from the hospital (post-test). The authors reported that "over 50 patients" participated in the self-medication program over an 18-month period. However, the results showed that 20 patients participated in the pretest and 79 in the post-test. Pretest data were obtained from patients admitted to the unit within 6 months prior to implementation of the self-medication program, and post-test data were obtained from patients who were admitted and discharged within 6 months after the program started. The results showed increases in patients' knowledge of name, dose, effects, and instructions between pre- and post-test, with the largest increase in the measure for medication effects. Measures for time and rationale of medication regimen decreased, but only by a small amount.

This article showed how patient education increased compliance and knowledge of medications so that patients could better care for themselves. It showed the responsiveness of the indicator to nursing care but was not linked directly to nursing care in nonacute care settings. Furthermore, this article did not test the validity or reliability of the self-medication to reducing risk of illness. The composition of the pre- and post-test sample is not described. Considering that the pretest sample was relatively small ($N = 20$), there may be confounding factors that account for the differences in knowledge of medication regimen. Additionally, there is no reliability or validity test of the assessment tool to determine if it is an appropriate tool to measure knowledge of medication regimen. Finally, there were no statistical tests performed to determine whether the differences between pre- and post-test were significant.

Debusk, R.F., N.H. Miller, H.R. Puerko, C.A. Dennis, R.J. Thomas, H.T. Lew, W.E. Berger, R.S. Heller, J.G. Rompf, D. Gee, H.C. Kraemer, A. Bandura, G. Ghandour, M. Clark, R.V. Shah, L. Fisher, and C.B. Taylor (1994). A case-management system for coronary risk factor modification after acute myocardial infarction. *Annals of Internal Medicine* 120(9): 721–9.

This study evaluated the efficacy of a physician-directed, nurse-managed, home-based case-management system for coronary risk factor modification compared to usual medical care. The case-management system (that is, the intervention group), derived from social learning theory, included interventions for smoking cessation, exercise training, and diet-drug therapy for hyperlipidemia. Intervention after discharge was implemented primarily through telephone and mail contact with patients in their homes. The sample of patients ($N = 585$; 65 percent of total) was drawn from the group of men and women age 70 years or younger who were hospitalized for acute myocardial infarction (AMI) in one of five Kaiser Permanente Medical Centers in the San Francisco Bay area between November 1988 and April 1991 (894 total). The sample was randomly assigned to intervention ($n = 293$) and control groups ($n = 292$). The results show that the smoking cessation rate, as measured by patients' self-report and biochemical confirmation, was significantly higher for the intervention group (70 percent) than it was for the control group (53 percent) at 12 months after AMI ($p = .03$). Functional capacity, expressed in METS or multiples of resting energy consumption, was used to assess exercise training. The intervention group showed significantly better functional capacities at 12 months compared to the usual care group (9.3 METS versus 8.4 METS; $p = .001$). Plasma

LDL cholesterol levels were also significantly lower for the intervention group (2.77 mmol/L) compared to the control group (3.41 mmol/L; $p = .001$). Although the authors noted that the study was unable to evaluate the long-term effectiveness of the intervention, they did report trends for lower reinfarction rates (3.4 percent versus 6.8 percent), but this difference was not statistically significant.

This study demonstrated that nurse-managed interventions for smoking cessation, exercise training, and diet/nutrition education can significantly lower risk factors for AMI. The long-term efficacy of the intervention for reducing the risk for reinfarction, however, was suggested but not confirmed by statistical analyses (that is, supports validity). The differences between the treatment and control groups suggested that the nursing interventions are responsive. Although the patients included in the study were identified from hospitalized patients, the interventions were implemented primarily in the home or outpatient setting, thus demonstrating applicability to nonacute care. Further testing must be done to determine the reliability and sensitivity of these interventions.

Erickson, H., and M.A. Swain (1990). Mobilizing self-care resources: a nursing intervention for hypertension. *Issues in Mental Health Nursing* 11: 217–35.

This study assessed the efficacy of a nursing intervention aimed at assisting the subject to contend with stressors that contribute to his or her hypertension. By doing so, according to modeling and role-modeling theory, subjects are able to mobilize internal and external self-care resources to contend with perceived stressors (or distressors) in a health and growth-directed manner. Subjects were told they could have up to an hour of the nurse researchers' time each week to discuss things that concerned or worried them and explore alternative ways to solve their problems. Ten subjects were placed in the treatment group, after written communication with clinics describing the project and asking for patient volunteers to participate in the project. The comparison group was identified in the same manner and matched to treatment group subjects on age and sex. Because treatment subjects were free to terminate from the study at any time, it was not possible to match also on the length of time in treatment. The comparison group was in treatment an average of 1.4 months longer than the experimental group. However, it is not clear from the article what determined the end-point for the comparison group. Blood pressure measurements (systolic and diastolic) were taken at the initial visit and at each subsequent visit. In addition, a Gleser-Gottschalk Word Adjective Checklist (GGWAC) was completed at the initial visit and presumably at each subsequent visit (although this is not explicitly stated in the article). The GGWAC is a 73-item survey that allows the researchers to score five subscales of feelings: active-happiness, tense-anxiousness, sad-depression, fatigue, and anger-hostility. Cornbach's alpha for internal consistency of each subscale was calculated and found to be acceptable for research (that is, all had alpha values greater than .80). Evidence of validity was found in three previous studies. After adjusting for entry systolic blood pressure values, analysis of covariance showed that the terminal systolic values differed significantly between the treatment and comparison group. Adjusted mean systolic blood pressures were 133.4 and 146.8 [F(1,17) = 20.9; p = .01] for the treatment and comparison groups, respectively. Adjusted mean diastolic blood pressures were also significantly different between the two groups, with values of 81.1 and 97.7 [F(1,17); p = .0003] at the end of the study for the treatment and comparison groups, respectively. Similarly, the two groups differed significantly with respect to the increase in feelings of active-happiness (U = 24.5; p = .05) and the decrease in feelings of tense-anxiousness (U = 12.5; p = .004). Additionally, the experimental group was less fatigued (U = 29.5; p = .11) and less sad and depressed (U = 27.5; p = .07), but the differences were not significant.

The results of this study supported the relationship between nursing interventions to improve patients' coping skills and a reduction in blood pressure, increased feelings of happiness, and decreased feelings of anxiousness. The limitations of this study included that subjects volunteered to participate in the study, subjects were not randomized into treatment and comparison groups, and the sample size was small. It is also curious that the comparison group remained in the study longer than the treatment group. The authors should also have found some way to quantify the treatment and given more detail on what was involved in the nursing intervention. However, the study is useful for demonstrating the validity of using coping skills to measure risk reduction and may be generalizable to other patient populations.

Graham, K.M., D.A. Pecoraro, M. Ventura, and C.C. Meyer (1993). Reducing the incidence of stomatitis using a quality assessment and improvement approach. *Cancer Nursing* 16(2): 117–22.

This study developed a protocol and patient teaching form for decreasing the incidence of stomatitis among patients receiving chemotherapy treatment. Prior to treatment, patients were given a teaching form with oral care instructions by nursing staff from the oncology unit at the Buffalo Veterans Administration Medical Center. The oncology unit consisted of 27 inpatient beds and an outpatient infusion room. A monitoring tool was also developed to determine if stomatitis developed and whether or not the protocol was followed and/or the patient complied with the oral care instructions. Itis assumed (but not clearly stated in the article) that this tool is completed each time the patient comes in for chemotherapy treatment. The outcome measure was the percent of patients with grade III stomatitis identified each month, where an average of 46 patients were treated each month (range 30–74). The total number of patients included in the study was 1,017 (all cases, no controls).

The findings show a trend toward a decreased percentage of patients with stomatitis over more than a 2-year period (data were collected from July 1989 to September 1991). The findings of this data support the validity of patient compliance with medication regimen as an indicator for risk reduction and the validity of management of symptoms of oral/nutritional status as an indicator for change in symptom severity. The limitations of this study are that tests of statistical significance were not conducted, and the reliability, responsiveness, and generalizability of these findings has not been determined.

McCloskey, J., and G. Bulechek (1995). Validation and coding of the NIC taxonomy structure. *Image: Journal of Nursing Scholarship* 27(1): 43–9.

The results of this study supported the face validity of the relationship between the quality or availability of nursing care and activity and exercise management, elimination management, immobility management, nutrition support, physical comfort promotion, self-care facilitation, electrolyte and acid-base management, drug management, neurologic management, perioperative care, respiratory management, skin and wound management, thermoregulation, tissue perfusion management, behavior therapy, cognitive therapy, communication enhancement, coping assistance, patient education, psychological comfort promotion, crisis management, risk management, childbearing care, life-span care, health system mediation, health system management, information management, crisis management, and risk management (abuse, delirium, delusion, dementia, environmental management, fall prevention, health screening, immunization administration, infection control, pressure ulcer prevention, radiation therapy management, and seizure management). The weakness of this study is that it is based on professional opinions and does not involve the clinical testing of the impact of nursing interventions on any of these areas.

Proos, M., Reiley, P., Eagan, J., Stengrevics, S., Castile, J., and Arian, D (1992). A study of the effects of self-medication on patients' knowledge of and compliance with their medication regimen. *Journal of Nursing Care Quality* Suppl: 18–26.

The purpose of this study was to determine if a self-medication program improved patient compliance with and knowledge of their medication regimen. The study was conducted on patients hospitalized in a major metropolitan teaching hospital. Upon admission, patients were assessed in terms of their eligibility for inclusion in the study (that is, was the patient oriented, without significant visual impairment, physically able to self-administer medications, and likely to be discharged home?). The group of eligible patients who consented to be in the study (N = 92) were randomized and assigned to treatment (self-medication program, n = 48) or control (structured teaching, n = 42) groups. There were no significant differences between the treatment and control groups on gender, mean age, mean number of medications, and mean number of days in study (hospitalized). During the inpatient stay, patients who were in the self-medication program underwent a teaching program administered by the primary nurse with written guidance and assistance from the hospital pharmacist and eventually self-administered their medications in the hospital. The structured teaching group received the same written information and individual counseling, but they did not self-administer their medications. At some point before medication information was received (pretest) and the time discharged from the hospital (post-test), patients were asked five questions pertaining to the knowledge of their medications. Both groups showed improvements between pre- and post-test scores, but the subjects in the self-medication group had significantly greater increases in all areas except for dosage than subjects in the structured teaching group. Compliance was measured one month after discharge from the hospital by counting the number of pills the patient took and dividing by the number of pills the patients should have taken as prescribed by the physician. While the compliance score of the self-medication group was higher (94.00) than the structure teaching group (90.05), the difference was not found to be significant.

This article demonstrated a link between self-medication and compliance, but not necessarily a link between compliance and risk reduction (that is, validity not demonstrated). In combination with Barry (1993), the results of this study show the reliability of tools used to measure effects of self care interventions. While the results were positive and there appears to be a strong link between nursing care and the knowledge and compliance measures used in this study, it is unclear whether these outcomes would be observed and how the intervention would be employed in a non-acute care setting.

Taylor, C.B., N. Houston-Miller, J.D. Killen, and R.F. DeBusk (1990). Smoking cessation after acute myocardial infarction: effects of a nurse-managed intervention. *Annals of Internal Medicine* 113(2): 118–23.

This study determined the effectiveness of a nurse-managed intervention to reduce smoking after acute myocardial infarction (AMI). Over a two-year period, research nurses interviewed eligible, hospitalized AMI patients from Kaiser Foundation hospitals in Redwood City, Santa Clara, Hayward, and San Jose, California. Patients who reported smoking cigarettes, cigarillos, or using any other form of tobacco in the 6 months preceding the AMI were recruited for study and randomized into treatment or control groups. The treatment group (n = 86) received the nurse-managed intervention, which incorporated principles of social learning theory and self-efficacy. It began one day after randomization, the first component taking place in the hospital. Nurses provided oral and written information about the dangers of smoking after AMI, benefits of not smoking, ways to cope with high-risk situations for smoking, and development of an action plan for smoking cessation. After discharge from the hospital, nurses initiated telephone contact with patients once per week for the first two to three weeks and then monthly for the next 4 months to determine whether the patient had relapsed or lost confidence in their ability to remain nonsmokers. No further intervention occurred after 6 months. The control group (n = 87) received usual care, which is to say that they received no specific instructions on how to stop smoking. The groups were similar along medical, smoking, and demographic characteristics, except that the usual care group drank significantly more than the treatment group ($p < .001$). One hundred thirty patients were followed up at 12 months after AMI to determine smoking status. Patients were considered nonsmokers if they stated they were not smoking, their carbon monoxide was less than 10 parts per million, and their serum thiocyanate was less than 110. The results showed that the smoking cessation rate was significantly higher for the treatment group (71 percent) than it was for the control group (45 percent; $p = .003$) one year after AMI. Furthermore, using a multiple logistic regression analysis, two predictors of smoking status at 12 months were identified—smoking at 3 weeks (odds ratio 22.7, CI 5.9 to 87.5) and self-efficacy (odds ratio 1.0, CI 1.0 to 1.1). Finally, the authors reported that there were no significant differences in cardiac event rates between the two groups at 12 months.

This study demonstrated a clear link between nonacute nursing care and outcome measures for smoking cessation and the responsiveness of smoking cessation to a nursing intervention. There did not appear to be any link between smoking status and risk reduction from the fact that there were no significant differences between the two groups in terms of cardiac events within 1 year after initial admission for AMI (that is, may not be a valid measure of risk reduction). Furthermore, reliability and generalizability of smoking cessation could not be confirmed from this article.

Wagner, E.H., A.Z. LaCroix, L. Grothaus, S.G. Leveille, J.A. Hecht, K. Artz, K. Odle, and D.M. Buchner (1994). Preventing disability and falls in older adults: a population-based randomized trial. *American Journal of Public Health* 84(11): 1800–6.

This article is important for demonstrating that a modest, one-time prevention program can have short-term health benefits. More specifically, the experimental nursing intervention was valid and responsive for preventing falls and injurious falls. It also indicated some success in getting people to exercise more. However, these results were based on self-reports, which may be biased, since they rely on patient recall. Further research will need to be conducted to confirm the reliability and responsiveness of the interventions for preventing falls and getting people to exercise regularly. (See section on Increase in Protective Factors for a description of this study.)

7. Increase in Protective Factors

Abraham, I.L., and S.J. Reel (1992). Cognitive nursing interventions with long-term care residents: effects on neurocognitive dimensions. *Archives of Psychiatric Nursing* VI (6): 356–65.

The purpose of this study was to determine whether nursing interventions would produce improvements in the cognitive functioning of nursing home residents. The sample consisted of 76 older adults residing in seven nursing homes who met sampling criteria specific to subjects' ability to participate in group interventions. Of these subjects, 30 participated in cognitive-behavioral groups, 29 in focused visual imagery groups, and 17 in education-discussion groups. There were 19, 15, and 8 left in each of the respective groups for the post-treatment data collection. Applying power tables from Kirk, the residual subsample sizes satisfied the requirements for detecting differences. A recently developed but psychometrically strong extension of the Mini-Mental State Exam was used to screen cognitive status and dementia. Three clinical nurse specialists with credentials and experience in respective treatment modalities conducted 24-week group interventions. Four trained interviewers, who were blinded to the treatment conditions to which subjects were assigned, were randomly assigned to each of the nursing homes. Data were collected according to a preestablished calendar 4 weeks before interventions, 8 and 20 weeks after the initiation of treatment, and 4 weeks after the conclusion of the interventions. In order to quantify the change in scores on cognitive parameters for subjects in a given treatment condition, a standardized index was derived. The results demonstrated that there were significant differences in the results achieved with the various interventions ($F (2,36) = 3.91$; $p = .05$). With main effects for the type of intervention on the Similarities ($F(2, 36) = 3.32$; $p < 5$), Mental Reversal ($F(2,36) = 3.59$; $p < .05$), and Writing ($F (2,36) = 3.58$; $p < 5$) portions of the score. Changes in all but one of the five categories of cognitive performance were identified.

The results of this study support the validity, sensitivity, and responsiveness of cognitive functioning as an indicator of level of functioning. In addition, the results of this study establish a link between the quality or availability of nursing care in nursing homes and level of cognitive functioning. The limitations of this study include the small sample size and the limited information presented about any other cognitive interventions that the subjects were receiving.

Anderson, B., J. Ho, J. Brackett, D. Finkelstein, and L. Laffel (1997). Parental involvement in diabetes management tasks: relationships to blood glucose monitoring adherence and metabolic control in young adolescents with insulin-dependent diabetes mellitus. *The Journal of Pediatrics* 130(2): 257–65.

This study identified parental behaviors that relate to adherence and metabolic control in a population of young adolescents with Insulin Dependent Diabetes Mellitus (IDDM). A cross-sectional design was used with a sample of 89 adolescents from a pediatric unit of the Joslin Diabetes Center in Boston, Massachusetts. Subjects were stratified into two age groups: (1) younger adolescents (10 to12 years old; $n = 51$) and (2) older adolescents (13 to15 years old; $n = 38$). There were no significant differences between the older and younger groups with respect to duration of diabetes, gender, parents' occupational or education status, number of daily insulin injections, or units of insulin per kilogram per day. During a regularly scheduled medical visit, demographic information and information about parental involvement in diabetes management were obtained. There were two measures of parental involvement in diabetes management tasks: (1) insulin injections and (2) blood glucose monitoring (BGM). For the former, families were asked who was usually (in the preceding month) responsible for five components of insulin injections: selecting dose, drawing up insulin, selecting the site, injecting the insulin, and supervising the injection. For the latter, four components were assessed: deciding when to check, checking (such as doing fingerstick), logging results, and parental awareness of results. For each component of both major tasks, families rated parental involvement on a scale of 1 to 4, with 1 indicating no parental involvement and 4 indicating maximum parental involvement. Reliability of this coding scheme was checked and revealed a 94 percent inter-rater reliability. Also at the clinic visit, the physician assessed the adolescent's adherence to diabetes management tasks by using a modified version of the Adherence Scale developed by Jacobson et al. (1990). Adherence was measured in the 3 to 4 months preceding the clinic visit with respect to the following areas of diabetes management: following a meal plan, amount of exercise, frequency of BGM, and insulin administration with use of a sliding scale. Glycemic control, which was the dependent variable, was measured by blood samples drawn at the time of the clinic visit, using total glycosolated hemoglobin counts. The results show that subjects in the younger age group checked their blood sugar concentrations significantly more often per day ($p < .007$) and had lower total glycosolated hemoglobin counts ($p < .02$) and had greater parental involvement with insulin injections ($p < .003$) than subjects in the older age group. Using multivariate analysis and controlling for various confounding factors, the authors found that parental involvement with either insulin injection or BGM did not predict glycemic control. However, significant predictors for adherence to BGM were Tanner stage of development ($p < .05$) and parental involvement in BGM ($p < .03$) and that frequency of BGM significantly predicted glycemic control ($p < .02$). The direct link between nursing care and patient compliance with treatment plans and involvement of caregivers is not explicitly stated, but general patient compliance to treatment regimens and self-care are considered areas of nursing practice. The context of the intervention, targeting caregiver involvement, and the results of the study (that is, better glycemic control) support the validity of the involvement of a primary caregiver as an indicator of increased protective factors, and the patient to treatment plans is an indicator of risk reduction. The reliability of these results was demonstrated by the fact that there was a 94 percent inter-rater reliability. The involvement also showed responsiveness; the children of less involved parents (older age group) had higher total glycosolated hemoglobin counts. It is unclear from this article, but it may be assumed that these findings are sensitive and generalizable

Coenen, A., P. Ryan, J. Sutton, E.C. Devine, H.H. Werley, and S. Kelber (1995). Use of the Nursing Minimum Data Set to describe nursing interventions for select nursing diagnoses and related factors in an acute care setting. *Nursing Diagnosis* 6(3): 108–14.

This study demonstrated the validity of symptom management/relief for pain and fluid and electrolyte status as indicators of change in symptom severity. In addition, it established the link between symptom management/relief for pain, fluid and electrolyte status, and injury prevention and the quality or availability of nursing care. (See the section on Changes in Symptom Severity for a description of this study.)

Olds, D.L., H. Kitzman, C.R. Henderson, C. Hanks, R. Cole, R. Tatelbaum, K.M. McConnochie, K. Sidora, D. W. Luckey, W. Shaver, K. Engelhardt, D. James, and K. Barnard (1997). Effect of prenatal and infancy home visitation by nurses on pregnancy outcomes, childhood injuries, and repeated childbearing. *Journal of the American Medical Association* 278(8): 644–53.

This study demonstrated that home nursing visits can lead to decreased healthcare use by reducing both the number of emergency room visits and hospital admission rates. The study also demonstrated that the availability of prenatal and postpartum home nursing care can lead to an increase in protective factors, resulting in a decrease in injuries to the child. The differences in the results achieved by the different treatment groups demonstrates the validity, sensitivity, and responsiveness of the number and appropriateness of emergency room visits, hospital admission rates, and a decrease in injuries as indicators of the quality or availability of nursing care. (See the section on Utilization of Services for a description of this study.)

Lange, M. (1996). The challenge of fall prevention in home care: a review of the literature. *Home Healthcare Nurse* 14(3): 198–206.

This article reviewed literature regarding falls and outlines elements for successful clinical nursing interventions that can be used to prevent falls, particularly among older adults. Falls among older adults are associated with approximately 18 percent of all restricted-activity days and play a big part in diminishing the quality of life. Older people suffer different types of injury from falls, but their response to injury and their ultimate outcome are quite different from those of younger patients. Secondary complications from falls may include immobility, hypothermia, deep vein thrombosis, stasis pneumonia, joint contractures, dehydration, urinary tract infections, and pressure ulcers. Specific risk factors for falls include a history of previous falls, health problems, a history of falling while performing activities of daily living, some degree of isolation in living arrangements, and being a woman over 75 years of age. Generally, risk factors are categorized into extrinsic and intrinsic factors. The extrinsic factors are related to the environment of the patient and include unstable furniture, shiny floors, poorly soled shoes, and dim lighting. Intrinsic factors are those related to the patient's health status, such as vision, hearing, balance, and medications. Wood and Cunningham (1992) reported that fall-prevention programs may reduce the number of falls, preventing injury and possibly death. A primary prevention program attempts to modify the environment to prevent falls, including making sure that walkways are in good repair, putting handrails on stairs, making steps slip-proof, and stapling down telephone and electrical cords (Jech 1992).

The article provided an important summary of the risk factors for falls and identified nursing interventions, particularly those that modify the home environment, that prevent falls from occurring. There is a tie to nursing in nonacute care settings, but the validity, reliability, responsiveness, and sensitivity of particular interventions was not provided in this article.

McCloskey, J., and G. Bulechek (1995). Validation and coding of the NIC taxonomy structure. *Image: Journal of Nursing Scholarship* 27(1): 43–9.

The results of this study support the face validity of the relationship between the quality or availability of nursing care and activity and exercise management, elimination management, immobility management, nutrition support, physical comfort promotion, self-care facilitation, electrolyte and acid-base management, drug management, neurologic management, perioperative care, respiratory management, skin and wound management, thermoregulation, tissue perfusion management, behavior therapy, cognitive therapy, communication enhancement, coping assistance, patient education, psychological comfort promotion, crisis management, risk management, childbearing care, life-span care, health system mediation, health system management, information management, crisis management, and risk management (abuse, delirium, delusion, dementia, environmental management, fall prevention, health screening, immunization administration, infection control, pressure ulcer prevention, radiation therapy management, and seizure management). The weakness of this study is that it is based on professional opinions and does not involve the clinical testing of the impact of nursing interventions on any of these areas. (See the section on Changes in Symptom Severity for a description of this study.)

Mittelman, M.S., S.H. Ferris, E. Shulman, G. Steinberg, and B. Levin (1996). A family intervention to delay nursing home placement of patients with Alzheimer disease: a randomized controlled trial. *Journal of the American Medical Association* 276(21): 1725–31.

The objective of this study was to determine the long-term effectiveness of comprehensive support and counseling for spouse-caregivers and families in postponing or preventing nursing home placement of patients with

Alzheimer disease (AD). Subjects were spouses of AD patients living at home at baseline and were primarily responsible for the care of the AD patient. Subjects were recruited over a 3 1/2-year period from among caregivers of patients at the New York University-Aging and Dementia Research Center. Subjects were randomized into treatment and control groups. The treatment consisted of three components: individual and family counseling sessions within the first 4 months after the caregiver was enrolled in the study; at the end of the 4 months, caregivers were required to participate in support groups that met weekly and continued indefinitely; and continuous availability of counselors to caregivers and families to help them deal with crises and the changing nature and severity of the patient's illness. The control group received regular services provided to families of patients with AD. They did not receive structured individual or family counseling sessions, and they were not required to join support groups. The treatment and control groups were found to be similar on most demographic and severity of dementia measures, except that there were significantly more female caregivers in the treatment group compared to the control group ($p = .02$). The results showed that patients in the treatment group remained at home significantly longer than those in the control group, using Breslow's test for equality of survival distribution stratified by caregiver sex ($p = .02$). Specifically, the intervention reduced the risk of nursing home placement between 2.5 and 5 times for patients with mild to moderate levels of dementia.

This study demonstrated a clear link between admission rates and nursing care in settings other than acute care, and showed how continuous available support and information can enable spouse-caregivers to withstand the difficulties of caring for AD patients and avoid nursing home placement. Like the Anderson article, it shows how the involvement of caregivers is a valid measure of increase in protective factors. Responsiveness of caregiver involvement is demonstrated by the differences between treatment and control groups. However, reliability, generalizability, and sensitivity were not tested in this study.

Olds, D., C.R. Henderson, H. Kitzman, and R. Cole (1995). Effects of prenatal and infancy nursing home visitation on surveillance of child maltreatment. *Pediatrics* 95(3): 365–72.

This study demonstrated that home nursing visits can lead to decreased healthcare utilization by reducing both the number of emergency room visits and hospital admission rates. The study also demonstrated that the availability of prenatal and postpartum home nursing care can lead to an increase in protective factors, resulting in a decrease in injuries to the child. The differences in the results achieved by the different treatment groups demonstrates the validity, sensitivity, and responsiveness of the number and appropriateness of emergency room visits, hospital admission rates, and a decrease in injuries as indicators of the quality or availability of nursing care. (See the section on Utilization of Services for a description of this study.)

Olds, D.L., J. Eckenrode, C.R. Henderson, H. Kitzman, J. Powers, R. Cole, K. Sidora, P. Morris, L.M. Pettitt, and D. Luckey (1997). Long-term effects of home visitation on maternal life course and child abuse and neglect: fifteen-year follow-up of a randomized trial. *Journal of the American Medical Association* 278(8): 637–43.

This study examined the long-term effects of a prenatal and early childhood home visitation program on child abuse and neglect and women's life course. This randomized trial was conducted in Elmira, New York, a semirural community. Of the 400 women enrolled in the program described in Olds (1995), 324 participated in a follow-up study when their children were 15 years old. Information about the women's use of welfare and number of subsequent children were collected via self-report; their arrests and convictions based on self-report and archived data from New York state; and verified reports of child abuse and neglect were abstracted from state records. During the 15-year follow-up period studied, the incidence of the women being identified as perpetrators of child abuse and neglect was .29 for the women who received home nursing visits during pregnancy and early childhood versus .54 for the other women ($p < .001$). Those who were unmarried and of low socioeconomic status at initial enrollment had an average of 1.3 subsequent births versus 1.6 among the comparison group ($p = .02$); 65 versus 37 months between children ($p = .001$); 60 versus 90 months for receiving aid to families with dependent children ($p = .005$); and 41 percent versus 73 percent for behavioral impairments due to use of alcohol and other drugs ($p = .03$), the incidence of arrests by self-report was .18 versus .58 ($p < .001$), and .16 versus .90 incidence of arrests disclosed by New York state records ($p < .001$).

This study demonstrated that home nursing visits to pregnant and postpartum women can lead to an increase in protective factors, resulting in a decrease in injuries and child abuse. The differences in the results achieved by the different treatment groups demonstrated the validity, sensitivity, and responsiveness of a decrease in injuries and child abuse as an indicator of the quality or availability of nursing care.

Olds, D.L., and H. Kitzman (1990). Can home visitation improve the health of women and children at environmental risk? *Pediatrics* 86(1): 108–16.

This study reviewed several randomized trials to determine the efficacy of home visitation programs for women or families that were at environmental risk for maternal and child health problems. Specifically, the trials reviewed focused on improving women's health-related behaviors during pregnancy, the birth weight and length of gestation of babies born to smokers and young adolescents, parents' interaction with their children, and children's developmental status. The study also focused on reducing the incidence of child abuse and neglect, childhood behavioral problems, emergency department visits and hospitalizations for injury, and unintended subsequent pregnancies. From the review, home visitation programs with the greatest chances for success had the following characteristics: they were based on ecological models; they were designed to address the ecology of the family during pregnancy and the early childbearing years with the nurse home visitors who established a therapeutic alliance with the families; and they targeted families at greater risk for maternal and child health problems by virtue of their poverty and lack of personal and social support. In the ecology model, the home visitors examined maternal and personal resources, social support, and stresses in the home, family, and community that can facilitate or interfere with optimal health-related behaviors during pregnancy or after childbirth. Forming a strong therapeutic alliance with the mother and her family is inherent in the ecological model. The strongest prenatal trial was the Elmira study (Olds et al. 1985, 1986), which showed that employing the ecological model resulted in significant improvements in birth weight and length of gestation. The Elmira, New York, study also contained a postnatal component, attempting to improve children's developmental accomplishments by teaching parents about factors that influence infant development and by promoting sensitive and growth-promoting caregiving. Significant differences were found between treatment and control groups on the number of stimulating toys in the home ($p < .01$) and the amount of restrictive or punitive behavior ($p < .05$). Finally, the Elmira study also tested the effects of nurse home visitation on child abuse and maltreatment. Among families at greatest sociodemographic risk for child abuse, the incidence of maltreatment increased to 19 percent in the control group, but remained relatively low (4 percent) for the treatment group ($p = .07$). The reliability of this finding was demonstrated in review of children's emergency department records. The Seattle study (Barnard et al. 1985) also demonstrated strength for a mental health home nursing visitation model in which the nurse fostered a therapeutic relationship with the mother in an attempt to enhance the mother's social competence. There were significant differences in favor of the mental health group in assessment of the mothers' teaching and qualities of the home environment. At age two, children of low-IQ mothers in the mental health group had Bayley motor development scores that were nine points higher than their counterparts in another home nursing model. Finally, in a study conducted in Washington, D.C. (Gutelius et al. 1972, 1977), showed that nurse-visited children displayed better diets, greater self-confidence, and fewer behavioral problems (such as toilet training and extreme shyness) as preschoolers. Their mothers were more involved in educationally stimulating activities with their children, used more appropriate methods of handling behavioral problems, and were more likely to continue their own education.

This study demonstrated the validity and responsiveness of home nursing interventions to improve environmental factors influencing maternal and child health, including injury prevention, and use of primary caregiver. It also demonstrated the validity and responsiveness of interventions that incorporated strong therapeutic alliances between mothers and families with the home-visiting nurse. As this review noted, additional studies must be conducted using the same models (as those described in the Elmira, Seattle, and Washington, D.C., studies) to confirm the reliability of the findings from these studies.

Pfaff, K.M., L.E. Johnson, P.J. Savage, and J.R. Kues (1997). Evaluation of an assessment tool for equipment management (ATEM) of home oxygen concentrators. *Respiratory Care* 42(6): 611–16.

The objective of this study was to assess clients' or caregivers' ability to accurately and safely manage home oxygen equipment and backup systems. Forms commonly used by home oxygen equipment providers were compared with the Assessment Tool for Equipment Management (ATEM) of home oxygen concentrators (HOC). The ATEM addresses standards for knowledge assessment recommended by the Joint Commission on Accreditation of Healthcare Organizations, including knowledge of liter flow, hours of daily use, oxygen safety and emergency procedures, equipment maintenance and storage, use of backup supplies, and response to equipment malfunction. Seventy subjects were recruited from five regional home care companies who were first-time users of HOC. Each subject was interviewed twice during a home visit by different people, once using ATEM and another time using the forms from the oxygen equipment company. Patients were randomized to determine which type of assessment tool would be used for the first interview. In general, the second interview took place about 3 days after the original interview, with the second interviewer blind to the results of the first interview. The results show that the company forms are less specific and contain less information than the ATEM. The company forms were also more subjective in their assessment of knowledge of proper management equipment. Furthermore, the ATEM identified high-risk knowledge deficits related to equipment management 16 times more often than the company forms ($p < .001$).

This article demonstrated a clear link between the equipment management indicator and nonacute care nursing practices. With the similar results of the two methods of assessing equipment knowledge, the authors have demonstrated that the reliability of equipment management methods for the area of increase in protective factors. By demonstrating the ability to respond to equipment malfunction and perform oxygen safety and emergency procedures, the study established the validity of equipment management as an indicator of increase in protective factors. The limitations of this study are that the sensitivity and responsiveness of the indicator was not tested. It is assumed that the overall findings may be applied to other areas where assessment of equipment management is applicable.

Wagner, E.H., A.Z. LaCroix, L. Grothaus, S.G. Leveille, J.A. Hecht, K. Artz, K. Odle, and D.M. Buchner (1994). Preventing disability and falls in older adults: a population-based randomized trial. *American Journal of Public Health* 84(11): 1800–6.

This study assessed a randomized, controlled trial of a multicomponent intervention program. The study sample was drawn from the population of HMO enrollees from the Group Health Cooperative of Puget Sound who were 65 years and older, ambulatory, and independent in activities of daily living. Of the 5,240 individuals identified for inclusion in the study, 1,559 (or

30 percent) completed a baseline questionnaire and were randomized into two treatment groups and one control group, using a 2:1:2 ratio. In the experimental intervention group (n = 635), patients visited with a trained nurse/educator who targeted their interventions for seniors who were physically inactive, drank alcohol to excess, had hazards in the home, used prescription drugs that increased risk for fall or mental impairment, or had uncorrected hearing or visual impairments. Follow-up phone calls and mailed reminders summarized the results of the visit, identifying risk factors and interventions for reducing the risk of falls. The second group was the nurse-visit only group (n = 317) in which patients received an invitation to attend a chronic disease prevention visit with a different set of nurses. The visit focused on assessment and counseling related to cardiovascular disease prevention (smoking, diet, hypertension control, and stress management), breast and cervical cancer detection, influenza vaccination, and seat belt use. The control group received usual care with no specific interventions. Data collection consisted of baseline assessment and follow-up surveys at 1 and 2 years after randomization. Ninety percent of the experimental and visit-only groups attended the nurse assessment visit. There were no significant differences at baseline between the groups on age, gender, race, income, education, restricted activity days, medical outcomes study physical functioning score, falls in the previous 12 months, and hospitalizations. The results showed that the experimental group reported three fewer restricted-activity days ($p < .05$), and 1.3 fewer bed disability days ($p < .01$). The experimental group also had a significantly smaller percentage of members who reported a fall in the first year follow-up (27.5 versus 36.8; $p < .01$), and smaller percentage of members who reported an injurious fall in the first-year follow-up (9.9 versus 14.5; $p < .01$) than the usual care group. The experimental group also exhibited more favorable health behaviors than the usual care group in terms of the percentage of members who exercised for more than 15 minutes 3 times per week, the number of blocks walked per week, and the percentage of members who sought home safety inspection. The favorable numbers, however, were only significant for the home inspection behavior, and were significantly different between the experimental group and the usual care group and between the experimental group and the visit-only group. The visit-only group had intermediate levels of most outcome variables with no significant differences between experimental and usual care groups.

This article demonstrated that a modest, one-time prevention program can have short-term health benefits. More specifically, the experimental nursing intervention was valid and responsive for preventing falls and injurious falls. It also indicated some success in getting people to exercise more. However, these results were based on self-reports, which may be biased since they rely on patient recall. Further research must be conducted to confirm the reliability and responsiveness of the interventions for preventing falls and getting people to exercise regularly.

8. Satisfaction with Quality of Life

Abraham, I.L., and S.J. Reel (1992). Cognitive nursing interventions with long-term care residents: effects on neurocognitive dimensions. *Archives of Psychiatric Nursing* VI (6): 356–65.

The purpose of this study was to determine whether nursing interventions would produce improvements in the cognitive functioning of nursing home residents. The sample consisted of 76 older adults residing in seven nursing homes who met sampling criteria specific to subjects' ability to participate in group interventions. Of these subjects, 30 participated in cognitive-behavioral groups, 29 in focused visual imagery groups, and 17 in education-discussion groups. There were 19, 15, and 8 left in each of the respective groups for the post-treatment data collection. Applying power tables from Kirk, the residual subsample sizes satisfied the requirements for detecting differences. A recently developed but psychometrically strong extension of the Mini-Mental State Exam was used to screen cognitive status and dementia. Three clinical nurse specialists with credentials and experience in respective treatment modalities conducted 24-week group interventions. Four trained interviewers, who were blinded to the treatment conditions to which subjects were assigned, were randomly assigned to each of the nursing homes. Data were collected according to a preestablished calendar 4 weeks before interventions, 8 and 20 weeks after the initiation of treatment, and 4 weeks after the conclusion of the interventions. In order to quantify the change in scores on cognitive parameters for subjects in a given treatment condition, a standardized index was derived. The results demonstrated that there were significant differences in the results achieved with the various interventions ($F(2,36) = 3.91$; $p = .05$). With main effects for the type of intervention on the Similarities ($F(2, 36) = 3.32$; $p < 5$), Mental Reversal ($F(2,36) = 3.59$; $p < .05$), and Writing ($F(2,36) = 3.58$; $p < 5$) portions of the score. Changes in all but one of the five categories of cognitive performance were identified.

The results of this study support the validity, sensitivity, and responsiveness of cognitive functioning as an indicator of level of functioning. In addition, the results of this study establish a link between the quality or availability of nursing care in nursing homes and level of cognitive functioning. The limitations of this study include the small sample size and the limited information presented about any other cognitive interventions that the subjects were receiving.

Baas, L.S., J.A. Fontana, and G. Bhat (1997). Relationship between self-care resources and the quality of life of persons with heart failure: a comparison of treatment groups. *Progress in Cardiovascular Nursing* 12(1): 25–38.

This study determined whether their was a relationship between patient self-care resources and quality of life. The study involved a convenience sample of 38 patients at their first, second, or third visit to the outpatient clinic. Data were collected via chart review and response to surveys. Subjects were recruited from a large heart failure and transplant treatment program at a Midwestern medical center. The inclusion criteria consisted of the appropriate diagnosis and symptom severity status, age of 18 years or older, and the ability to read and write English. Exclusion criteria consisted of the presence of a cognitive or emotional disorder that would impede the person's ability to complete the surveys accurately. The patients completed demographic information, a Self-Care Resources Inventory, Human Activity Profile, Index of Well-Being, Short Form-36 Health Survey, and the Minnesota Living with Heart Failure Questionnaire. The chart review was conducted to determine the patients' diagnostic study results, proposed treatment plans, and the course of their illness. The correlation matrix revealed relationships among the global and health related measures of quality of life and self-care, physical and emotional symptoms, and activity for all 38 patients. Upon performing a regression analysis, it was determined that the self-care measures accounted for 38 percent of the variance in global quality of life as measured by the Index of Well-Being ($F = 20.15$, df 1,36, $p < .0001$).

The results of this study support the validity, reliability, and responsiveness of self-efficacy as an indicator of quality of well-being. The results are generalizable across nonacute care settings. The limitations of this study include the small sample size and the lack of a direct link to nursing care.

Baradell, J.G. (1995). Clinical outcomes and satisfaction of patients of clinical nurse specialists in psychiatric- mental health nursing. *Archives of Psychiatric Nursing* IX(5): 240–50.

The results of this study demonstrated the relationship between symptom management/relief cognition, psychological/neurological/cognitive functioning, communication, satisfaction with social functioning, satisfaction with role functioning, satisfaction with family coping, and satisfaction with quality of care rendered and the quality or availability of nursing care. (See the section on Changes in Symptom Severity for a description of this study.)

Bertero, C., Eriksson, B.E., and A.C. Ek (1997). A substantive theory of quality of life of adults with chronic leukemia. *International Journal of Nursing Studies* 34(1): 9–16.

This study determined what patients with leukemia considered to be the components of quality of life. The data were collected through taped interviews of patients. Criteria for selecting subjects were that they were adults suffering from chronic leukemia and registered as patients at a county hospital. There were 15 interviewees, 6 females and 9 males from 39 to 82 years of age. The interview guide approach was used and interviews were 25 to 60 minutes in length. The grounded theory method was used in this study. Data were analyzed using constant comparative methods; each word, line, phrase, and sentence was transcribed, reviewed, and coded. Satisfaction with quality of life was found to be related to self-esteem, interpersonal relationships, ability to perform roles in life, and social ability.

This study determined that self-esteem, interpersonal relationships, ability to perform roles in life, and social ability are valid indicators of quality of life. Limitations of this study were no direct link to nursing care; the study was performed in an acute care setting; and the reliability, responsiveness, and sensitivity of the indicators were not assessed.

Campbell, J.M. (1992). Treating depression in well older adults: use of diaries in cognitive therapy. *Issues in Mental Health Nursing* 13: 19–29.

The purpose of this study was to determine whether nurses could identify maladaptive depression in well, older adults and whether nursing intervention strategies made a significant difference in levels of depression in the well elderly. A nonprobability sample was selected from residents of two city-owned and two privately owned high-rise apartments for low-income, well, elderly persons. The group identified as depressed consisted of 80 women and 23 men ages 64 to 82. All of the subjects were diagnosed with nonsuicidal, nonpsychotic depression based on the criteria of the Diagnostic and *Statistical Manual of Mental Disorder, 3rd edition* (DSM-III-R). The nurses on staff in the four buildings were asked to use the DSM-III-R to identify 50 residents per building who were in their judgment depressed. One hundred and three residents who met the established criteria agreed to participate in the study. Subjects were assigned to three groups stratified by random sample according to gender, which resulted in equal gender distributions in each group. Group 1 received planned nursing interventions per a protocol that was based on cognitive therapy techniques, Group 2 received no intervention, and Group 3 received group classes and practice on crafts, but no specific treatment from nurses in order to rule out the Hawthorne effect. Study participants were informed of the study's purpose, the time frame, expectations, and the nurses' role. Nurses were given training on the use of the DSM-III-R, and the protocols planned for nursing intervention strategies. Subjects in the intervention group received individual therapy from an assigned nurse for 8 weeks, with two 1-hour interventions per week. The subjects were seen privately in common rooms of the housing units. One hundred and twelve individuals were identified as depressed, instead of the originally planned 200 participants. Of the 112, 103 were identified as being depressed by scoring at least in the moderately depressed range. The Zung Self-Rating Depression Scale (SRDS) was used to validate the ability of the nurses to identify depressed individuals. Their results were validated with 92 percent accuracy. At the conclusion of the nursing intervention, all of the individuals in the experimental group achieved Zung SRDS scores indicating mild or no depression, while the individuals in the nonintervention groups showed no changes from the original scores that demonstrated moderate to severe depression. The difference between the scores before and after the nursing intervention were statistically significant ($t = 3.83$; $p > 1$). There was also a significant difference between the median scores of the subjects in the craft group and in the experimental group (Mann-Whitney $U = 27$; $p > .05$).

The results of this study support the validity, sensitivity, and responsiveness of management/relief of cognitive symptoms as an indicator of change in symptom severity. Furthermore, the results of the study demonstrate a link between the quality or availability of nursing interventions in a nonacute care setting and the severity of patients' cognitive symptoms.

Ferrell, B.R., C. Wisdom, and C. Wenzl (1989). Quality of life as an outcome variable in the management of cancer pain. *Cancer* 63: 2321–7.

This study tested the validity and reliability of a quality assessment tool, which may be used as an outcome measure of pain management interventions. The City of Hope Medical Center Quality of Life Survey is a multidimensional instrument, including measures for psychological well-being, physical well-being, general symptom control, specific symptom control, and social support. There were three study groups: one for cancer patients with pain, one for cancer patients without pain, and one for patients without cancer. Fifty subjects were identified for each group from oncology units of the Mercy Health Center and Presbyterian Hospital in Oklahoma City, Oklahoma. Although the authors investigated age, gender, ethnicity, time since cancer diagnosis, and other illnesses of the subjects, no tests of significance were performed to determine if there were significant differences among the groups along these variables. Data for the study were gathered during an interview with the patient, conducted by two master's-level oncology nurses. The results indicate that the quality of life instrument had test–retest reliability (reliability coefficient of > .60 as reported in previous study), internal consistency (*r* values > =.65 using Cronbach's alpha), and inter-rater reliability using a pain assessment tool and the Karnofsky rating for functional performance (*r* values .94 and .82, respectively, using Person product moment correlation). In addition, the instrument demonstrated content validity (content validity index 0.90) and construct validity, supporting psychological well-being, worry, and nutrition.

In this study, there was no test of the a nursing intervention, but pain management is considered within the domain of nursing care. This study does demonstrate validity and reliability of a quality of life tool designed to assess the effectiveness of pain management programs. It is unclear whether this tool may be generalizable to other clinical conditions.

Grady, K.L., A. Jalowiec, C. White-Williams, R. Pifarre, J.K. Kirklin, R.C. Bourge, and M.R. Costanzo (1995). Predictors of quality of life in patients with advanced heart failure awaiting transplantation. *Journal of Heart and Lung Transplantation* 14(1): 2–10.

This study assessed life satisfaction in multiple areas; examined correlations between satisfaction and demographic, physiologic, and psychosocial variables; and identified the predictors of quality of life in patients with end-stage heart disease awaiting transplantation. Data were collected from a convenience sample of 359 English-speaking patients from Loyola University Medical Center and University of Alabama Medical Center who were awaiting heart transplantation. Patient age ranged from 18 to 70 years of age. Eight instruments were used to gather data from the patients: the Quality of Life Index, the Heart Transplantation Symptom Checklist, the Sickness Impact Profile, the Heart Transplant Stressor Scale, the Jaloweiec Coping Scale, The Heart Transplant Intervention Scale, the Social Support Index, and the Rating Question Form. Total subscale scores were derived for each tool, and the data were analyzed using descriptive statistics, Pearsons correlations, and stepwise multiple regression analysis. Limitations to regression analysis and violation of assumptions of regression were examined. The level of significance was set at 0.05. Significant correlation between overall life satisfaction and older age ($r = .13$; $p = .008$), a lower NYHA functional classification ($r = .16$; $p = .001$), overall functional disability ($r = .42$; $p < .0001$), symptom distress ($r = .44$; $p < .0001$), stress and coping ($r = .49$; $p < .0001$), providing information for self efficacy ($r = .19$; $p < .0001$), a better health perception ($r = .40$; $p < .0001$), and greater expectation of transplant success ($r = .27$; $p < .0001$).

The results of this study supported the validity, reliability, and responsiveness of physical functional status, social functional status, symptom distress, stress/coping, and self-efficacy as indicators of satisfaction with quality of life. The limitations of this study were the lack of a direct link to nursing care or a particular health care setting.

Keckeisen, M.E., and A.M. Nyamathi (1990). Coping and adjustment to illness in the acute myocardial infarction patient. *Journal of Cardiovascular Nursing* 5(1): 25–33.

In this study, the authors examined the coping strategies of acute myocardial infarction (MI) patients one month following discharge from the hospital. The hypothesis being tested was that there is a correlational relationship between an acute myocardial infarction patient's coping style (as determined by the ratio of problem-to and emotion-focused coping strategies) and the patient's psychological, social, and physiologic adjustment. Thirty acute MI patients from one of two participating medical centers participated in the study. Most were older than 50 years (77 percent) male (83 percent), and Caucasian (73 percent). More than half were married and employed prior to MI and nearly all were well-educated with a relatively high index of social class. Subjects were visited an average of 24 days after discharge at which time three tools were used to assess coping strategies. One was the Jalowiec Coping Scale (JSC), which assessed problem- and emotion-focused coping strategies. Reliability of the JSC was .85 for problem-focused and .47 for the emotion-focused subscales. The second tool was the Psychological Distress and the Social Environment subscales of the Psychosocial Adjustment to Illness Scale (PAIS-SR). This was assessed the degree to which patients made psychological and social adjustments. Internal consistency in this study was .83 for the psychological and .88 for the social environment subscales. Finally, the Physiological Symptom Subscale (PSS) of the Spousal Coping Instrument (SCI) measured physiological well-being and assessed the degree to which an individual responds to the MI. In particular, adaptive outcomes, such as sleep, chest pains, and fatigue were assessed. The results showed that individuals who used more problem-focused coping than emotion-focused coping had better social ($p < .005$) and psychological adjustment ($p < .05$). Further, individuals who had more physiological symptoms were found to have poorer psychological adjustment.

Although this study did not test the impact of a nursing intervention, there may be a weak link to nursing care in that nursing interventions may make use of these results in developing patient education tools or discharge planning protocols. There was also a weak link to the nonacute care setting in that the patients were visited in their homes to assess their coping skills. This study supported the validity of patient coping/burden/stress as an indicator for patient satisfaction with quality of life. Additionally, the tools used to measure coping skills were, with one exception, internally consistent, supporting reliability of the indicator.

Kuiper, R., and A.M. Nyamathi (1991). Stressors and coping strategies of patients with automatic implantable cardioverter defibrillators. *Journal of Cardiovascular Nursing* 5(3): 65–76.

This study identified the stressors, perceptions, and coping strategies of patients living with automatic implantable cardioverter defibrillators (AICD). This device is a form of therapy for persons who are at risk for sudden cardiac death and is designed to continuously monitor the electrical activity of the heart, to recognize ventricular tachycardia and fibrillation, and to deliver corrective defibrillatory shocks promptly when necessary. Twenty subjects (out of 35 possible subjects) participated in this study. In this descriptive study, medical and demographic information were recorded, the Jaloweic Coping Scale was used to assess problem-to and emotion-focused coping strategies, and a structured interview was conducted to elicit specific sources of stress and coping strategies for later content analysis. An interview guide was the basis on which the interviews were conducted. It contained 17 semistructure questions regarding stress and coping strategies. They explored activities of daily living, social activities, occupational activities, ambiguity and predictability of device discharge, role changes at home and work, changes in dependency needs, fear of being alone, social supports, relationships with others, past and future considerations, knowledge of deficits, and advice for other potential AICD patients. The typical AICD patient had been living with the device for 8.75 months, was male, married, Caucasian, educated past high school, Protestant, and working as a professional, homemaker, or manual laborer. The results show that patients use a mixture of problem-focused and emotion-focused coping strategies in the physical, psychological, and social areas. The optimistic coping style, however, facilitated coping most effectively. The mean use and mean effectiveness scores from the JCS were highest (1.7 and 1.5, respectively). The content analysis revealed that the frequency of perceptions of adjustment to stress fell into three major categories: physical ($n = 150$), psychological ($n = 135$), and social adjustments ($n = 138$).

This study, which was a descriptive study without treatment and control groups, supported the validity of the patient coping/burden/stress indicator for patient satisfaction with quality of life. However, links to nursing and practice in nonacute care settings were weak, as they were not specifically used, but they had implications for nursing practice in nonacute care settings. Additionally, this study did not confirm reliability, sensitivity, or responsiveness of the indicator for patient satisfaction with quality of life.

Lok, P. (1996). Stressors, coping mechanisms, and quality of life among dialysis patients in Australia. *Journal of Advanced Nursing* 23: 873–81.

This study determined what, if any, stressors and coping mechanisms are related to quality of life in dialysis patients. A questionnaire survey was conducted on patients in two dialysis centers in Sydney, Australia. A total of 111 patients receiving either of two types of dialysis at the participating centers was invited to participate in the study; they were given a cover letter explaining the purpose and design of the study, a consent form, and the questionnaire. Self-addressed stamped envelopes were provided for return of the study. Sixty-four of the patients (58 percent) returned completed questionnaires and consent forms. The questionnaire included Baldree's heamodialysis stressor scale for the measurement of stressors, Jalowiec and Powers' coping behaviors scale for measurement of coping mechanisms, and Padilla's quality of life index for measurement of the quality of life. The data were grouped into six groups: sociodemographic variables, problem-oriented coping score, affective-oriented coping score, physiologic stressor score, psychologic stressor score, and quality of life. Cronbach alphas were calculated to establish the reliability of the items in the questionnaire, and correlation coefficients were calculated to assess the degrees of association between the variables. All stressor items had a Cronbach alpha of 0.79, coping methods 0.86, and quality of life 0.71. The total questionnaire had a Cronbach alpha of 0.80. In the heamodialysis group, total stressor score was significantly correlated with quality of life ($r = .38$; $p < .05$) and coping methods ($r = .26$; $p < .05$). In the CAPD group, the total stressor score was negatively correlated with quality of life (.54; $p < .05$) and positively correlated with the coping score (.39; $p < .05$). Problem-solving coping methods were positively correlated with total quality of life in both groups, hemodialysis ($r = .39$; $p < .01$), and CAPD ($r = .48$; $p < .01$). The length of time on dialysis was related to the stressor scores but not the coping scores. The subjects ranked physical limitations as the number one stressor.

The results of this study demonstrated that stress, coping, and physical limitations/role functioning are valid, reliable indicators of quality of life. The limitations of this study were that there is no direct link to nursing care, and the sensitivity and responsiveness of the indicators have not been tested. The results do appear to be generalizable to all nonacute care settings; however, their generalizability was not tested.

Lowry, L., J. Saeger, and S. Barnett (1997). Client satisfaction with prenatal care and pregnancy outcomes. *Outcomes Management for Nursing Practice* 1(1): 29–35.

The purpose of this study was to determine whether nursing case management improved pregnancy outcomes and client satisfaction for pregnant women of low socioeconomic status. Two initiatives were implemented in the state of Florida. One was an improved Pregnancy Outcome Program (IPOP) delivered through the Human Resource Service County Public Health Clinics, and the other was a multidisciplinary ambulatory health care center for women and children (MDC). the IPOP clinic utilized advanced practice nurses (APNs) to deliver care in conjunction with an attending obstetrician on call fore obstetric or medical problems. The MDC utilized case management Registered Nurses (Rns) and APNs to serve as case managers for clients who received care from a team made up of Rns, APNs, obstetricians, gynecologists, social workers, nutrition counselors, and health educators. The first 62 pregnant clients from each clinic who were English-speaking, literate, and had given voluntary consent were invited to participate in the study during the fall of 1994. Clients with three or more clinic visits were asked to complete the Risser Patient Satisfaction Scale, developed to measure patient attitudes toward nurses and nursing care in ambulatory clinic settings. A new subscale of 6 items measuring factors related to setting was added to the Raiser instrument for the purposes of this study. The new subscale and the other three Risser scales were pilot tested on 30 of the pregnant clients, 15 from each clinic. Alpha coefficients for the pre and post tests were .79 and .74 , respectively. Test–retest reliability was calculated yielding an overall Pearson correlation coefficient of .86. Independent sample *t*-tests of means calculated for technical skill, teaching, interpersonal relationships, and setting indicated significant differences between treatment settings. Clients from the MDC group were more likely to agree with positive statements about nurses technical skill, teaching, and interpersonal relationships than were those from the PHC. There were no significant differences in health care outcomes between the two groups.

This study demonstrates the sensitivity, reliability, and responsiveness of satisfaction with quality of care rendered, and satisfaction with communication as indicators of satisfaction with quality of care. In addition, the study establishes a link between the quality or availability of nursing care in an outpatient setting, and patient satisfaction.

McCloskey, J., and G. Bulechek (1995). Validation and coding of the NIC taxonomy structure. *Image: Journal of Nursing Scholarship* 27(1): 43–9.

The results of this study support the face validity of the relationship between the quality or availability of nursing care and activity and exercise management, elimination management, immobility management, nutrition support, physical comfort promotion, self-care facilitation, electrolyte and acid-base management, drug management, neurologic management, perioperative care, respiratory management, skin and wound management, thermoregulation, tissue perfusion management, behavior therapy, cognitive therapy, communication enhancement, coping assistance, patient education, psychological comfort promotion, crisis management, risk management, childbearing care, life-span care, health system mediation, health system management, information management, crisis management, and risk management (abuse, delirium, delusion, dementia, environmental management, fall prevention, health screening, immunization administration, infection control, pressure ulcer prevention, radiation therapy management, and seizure management). The weakness of this study is that it is based on professional opinions and does not involve the clinical testing of the impact of nursing interventions on any of these areas. (See the section on Changes in Symptom Severity for a description of this study.)

Miakowski, C., and S.L. Dibble (1995). The problem of pain in outpatients with breast cancer. *Oncology Nursing Forum* 22(2): 791–9.

This study evaluated the effects of pain on the patient's performance of activities of daily living and satisfaction with quality of life. This was a descriptive correlational study involving a convenience sample of 97 outpatients actively being treated for breast cancer. The patients were adults who were able to read, write, and understand English. They were receiving certain types of outpatient cancer therapy and had a Karnofsky Performance Scale score of at least 50. Information was collected using a demographic questionnaire, a cancer pain questionnaire, the short-form Profile of Mood States (POMS), and the Multidimensional Quality of Life Scale-Cancer (MQOLA-CA2). After informed consent was obtained, all of the subjects were asked to complete the demographic questionnaire, KPS, POMS, and MQOLS-CA and to report whether they had experienced cancer-related pain in the past month. Independent student t-tests or chi-square analyses were performed to determine differences in sample characteristics, POMS scores, and MQOLS-CA scores between patients with and without cancer-related pain. Forty-seven percent of the patients with breast cancer reported experiencing cancer-related pain, and those patients had significantly lower scores on the quality of life measures ($t = 2.5$; $p < .01$) and significantly higher scores on the mood disturbance measures.

The results of this study support the validity and responsiveness of physical comfort/pain as an indicator of quality of well-being. Limitations of the study include the lack of a direct link to nursing care, and failure to assess the sensitivity of the relationship between pain and quality of well-being.

Paykel, E.S., S.P. Mangen, J.H. Griffith, and T.P. Burns (1982). Community psychiatric nursing for neurotic patients: a controlled trial. *British Journal of Psychiatry* 140: 573–81.

This study determined whether there was a difference in outcomes for patients receiving routine outpatient psychiatric care as opposed to those receiving home visits by psychiatric nurses. The nursing was based at

Springfield Hospital, London, a psychiatric hospital serving a local catchment area of 350,000. Outpatient clinics were held at several large hospital clinics and two smaller clinics in the London area. Eight full-time, psychiatric nurses were involved in the study. They worked in coordination with 10 catchment area teams, and in most cases they worked exclusively with one team. The sample consisted of patients being discharged from the hospital or having already completed 6 months of outpatient treatment. All subjects had International Classification of Diseases, ninth edition (ICD-9) diagnoses of neuroses, unipolar affective psychoses, or anankastic, hysterical, or asthenic personality disorders. All subjects were determined by the treatment team to be in need of at least 6 months of further follow-up care. All outpatient clinic attendees and impending hospital/day hospital discharges were screened for inclusion in the study. After initial assessment, suitable subjects were randomly assigned to one of the two treatment groups using a minimization procedure, which allowed matching on 14 demographic, diagnostic, history, and current rating variables. Treatment was continued for up to 18 months, and subjects who completed less than 6 months of treatment were dropped from the study. Contacts with the nurse and the precise nature of those contacts were as clinically indicated. Assessments were conducted by the research sociologist and psychologist not involved in the treatment. These took place initially and at 6-month intervals until the 18th month. Symptom assessments were made using the Clinical Interview for Depression, the Raskin Three Area Depression Scale, and the Covi Three Area Anxiety Scale. Social adjustment was assessed using the Social Adjustment Scale. Satisfaction was assessed at each interview with the patient and relative on a number of specific and global aspects. In addition, at the end of 18 months, the client completed a self-report questionnaire for consumer satisfaction. A reliability study between the two raters, on the interview symptom ratings and the Social Adjustment Scale, showed mean correlations of .82 and .85, respectively. A total of 99 patients were included in the main study sample. Seventy-one patients completed a full 18 months, with 36 in community psychiatric nursing and 35 in outpatient care. No differences were found in the effectiveness of the two modes of treatment on symptoms, social adjustment, or family burden. Community psychiatric resulted in a reduction in outpatient contacts with psychiatrists and other staff, a slight increase in contacts with general practitioners for prescriptions, and an improvement in patient satisfaction. A total of 46 percent of the group receiving community psychiatric care and 72 percent of the group receiving routine outpatient care was still receiving psychiatric care at the conclusion of 18 months of treatment. While the differences in overall patient satisfaction were not statistically significant, there was a statistically significant difference in the patients' satisfaction with the quality of care received $< .05$ and communication $< .05$, with the patients receiving psychiatric nursing care being more satisfied than those receiving routine outpatient care.

This study supported the validity, reliability, sensitivity, and responsiveness of patient satisfaction with quality of care rendered and patient satisfaction with communication as indicators of patient satisfaction. In addition, this study established a link between the quality or availability of nursing care in a community care setting and patient satisfaction with communication and patient satisfaction with quality of care rendered. The limitations of this study included the small sample size, the lack of information about potential confounding factors, and the lack of detailed information about the content of the patient satisfaction tools.

Peruselli, C., E. Paci, P. Francheschi, T. Legori, and F. Mannucci (1997). Outcome evaluation in a home palliative care service. *Journal of Pain and Symptom Management* 113(3): 158–65.

The largest improvement in symptoms secondary to quality nursing care was seen in the pain, functional, and psychological subscales. These results demonstrated that home nursing care can decrease the severity of pain and the psychological and functional symptoms experienced by patients. The results also showed that the severity of these symptoms changes and is measurable over time. These results should be generalizable to other nonacute care settings. (See section on Changes in Symptom Severity for a description of this study.)

Szabo, E., H. Moody, T. Hamilton, C. Ang, C. Kovithavongs, and C. Kjellstrand (1997). Choice of treatment improves quality of life: a study on patients undergoing dialysis. *Archives of Internal Medicine* 157: 1352–6.

This study compared the quality of life in persons who freely chose continuous ambulatory peritoneal dialysis (CAPD) and those who have been forced to undergo CAPD. The study involved retrospective chart review and administration of questionnaires. Historically, patients at a university hospital were able to choose between hemodialysis and CAPD. When the hemodialysis program became full, patients in need of dialysis had to have CAPD. Forty-four patients were studied during the period of choice, and the results were compared to the results of 45 patients who were studied during the period of no choice. There were no significant demographic differences between the two groups nor were there significantly different results in their health status or response to CAPD. A retrospective review of the patients' medical records was performed to determine their health status and response to treatment. Quality of life was determined by interviewing patients using a questionnaire that rated them on seven scales that are used to assess quality of life components. Four scales measured psychological well-being, the Bradburn Affect Scale, Mental Health Scale, Campbell Life Satisfaction Scale, and Perceived Health Scale. Three scales measured mainly physical well-being, the Karnofsky Scale, an activity scale, and a 20-item physical symptoms scale. The patients' desire for treatment change was also scored. The results were analyzed using the Statview 4.01 program. An analysis of variance, a Student *t*-test, and Fisher exact probability test were used in the statistical analysis. A $p < .05$ was regarded as significant. The patients undergoing CAPD in the no-choice group had a lower score than the choice group in four of the seven quality of life scales. The Mental Health Scale mean score was 18.4 compared to 15.5, and the patients ranking highest on the Mental Health Scale decreased from 33 percent to 18 percent, while those ranking lowest increased from 2 percent to 14 percent. The Bradburn Affect Scale score was +0.7 in the choice group compared with –0.3 in the no-choice group.

This study suggests that patient involvement in the treatment plan/strength of the therapeutic alliance is a valid indicator of patient satisfaction with quality of life. A limitation of this study is that it was not directly linked to nursing interventions. However, nurses have the ability to involve patients in their treatment decisions regardless of the setting.

Wallhagen, M.I., and M. Brod (1997). Perceived control and well-being in Parkinson's disease. *Western Journal of Nursing Research* 19(1): 11–31.

This study analyzed the impact of the patient's control over symptoms on patient and caregiver well-being and caregiver burden. One hundred and one Parkinson's disease patients, recruited for a larger study on stress and coping in Parkinson's disease also participated in this study. Patients were considered to be eligible for the study if they had a diagnosis of Parkinson's disease for more than 1 year, were not demented, were 60 years of age or older, resided in the community, and were without any other preexisting chronic illness. Sixty-nine of the patients had spouse caregivers, and 45 of these participated in a spouse caregiver portion of the study. All of the patients were interviewed twice at baseline in person, for approximately 1 hour and again at a 1-year follow-up telephone interview lasting approximately 20 minutes. Spouses of the patients were mailed a questionnaire at the time of the 1-year follow-up interview. Well-being was assessed using the Medical Outcomes Study Mental Health Index (MOS). In addition to the MOS, caregivers were mailed the Care Giver Burden Interview (CBI). Results for both groups were analyzed using bivariate correlational analyses. Regression analysis was used to assess the association between patients' perceived control over the symptoms and disease progression and the outcome variables of patient well-being and caregiver well-being and burden while controlling for the patients' perceived disease severity. A significant relationship was found between patient perception of control over symptoms and patient well-being ($r = .22$; $p = .026$), caregiver well-being ($r = 33$; $p = .027$), and caregiver burden ($r = .30$; $p = .047$). Results of the regression analysis demonstrated that perceived control over symptoms remained significantly associated with patient well-being ($B = 0.19$; $p = .05$), caregiver well-being ($B = 0.33$; $p = .029$), and caregiver burden ($B = -0.29$; $p = .03$).

The results of this study supported the validity, reliability, and responsiveness of patient efficacy as an indicator of patient satisfaction with quality of life.

Wyatt, G., M.E. Kurtz, L.L. Friedman, B. Given, and C.W. Given (1996). Preliminary testing of the Long-Term Quality of Life (LTQL) instrument for female cancer survivors. *Journal of Nursing Measurement* 4(2):153–70.

In this study, the investigators developed and tested an instrument to measure quality of life in long-term female cancer survivors. The study built on previous work by Grant and associates (1992), Ferrell (1993), and Dow et al. (1996). Focus groups were used to identify all potential items that should be included in the tool (i.e., covering the areas of interest and concern among the survivors). The study also sought to refine and strengthen spiritual/existential domains of quality of life. After four focus group discussions took place, a 67-item LTQL survey instrument was created, assessing the following content areas: eating habits, body image, apparel, pain, exercise, change in senses, change in social support, desire to be of service to others, relationships with healthcare providers, susceptibility to cancer, change in perception of health and illness, spiritual guidance for health decisions, and change in philosophical view of life. The survey and additional CaRES survey and demographic questions were mailed to 350 female cancer survivors, identified from the tumor registry of a Michigan hospital. The CaRES tool was used to validate the tool and measures five domains of quality of life: physical, psychosocial, medical interaction, marital, and sexual. This tool has been used for other cancer survivors, with demonstrated validity and reliability. In a factor analysis, the 67 items were reduced to an improved set of 39 and resulted in four factors, accounting for 53 percent of the total variance. The four factors were somatic concerns, philosophical/spiritual view of life, fitness, and social support. Internal consistency for the four subscales using Cronbach's alpha, were from .87 to .92 and were congruent with Ferrell's theoretical domains of quality of life. Content validity was supported through inter-rater agreement of subscale items. Significant correlations between the LTQL and the CaRES support the concurrent validity of the LTQL. In particular, the somatic factor was significantly correlated to all of the CaRES domains ($p < .002$) and the fitness scale was correlated with the physical domain of the CaRES instrument ($p < .002$).

This study supported the validity and reliability of satisfaction with social functioning and patient comfort as indicators for patient satisfaction with quality of life. The LTQL supported the validity and reliability of other indicators of satisfaction with quality of life, not being analyzed in the scientific merit of the indicators, including philosophical or spiritual view of life and fitness. This study, like many other studies in this area, was not specifically linked to nursing care or care in nonacute care settings, but implied that the tool could be used on patients receiving care from nurses in nonacute care settings. Additionally, this study was not designed to determine the sensitivity or responsiveness of these indicators, and generalizability cannot be inferred from this study.

APPENDIX C

References Used to Identify Nursing Quality Indicators

This appendix includes resources utilized in the initial identification of the most commonly cited indicators with an empirical or theoretical link to the eight areas identified by ANA and the availability or quality of nursing care.

The first section lists databases, tools/instruments, and resources that were included in the review. The second section presents the additional research-based articles and academic publications that contained references to quality care, quality indicators, nursing care, and patient outcomes.

Databases, Tools, Instruments, and Other Resources

Adult Asthma QoL Questionnaire (AQLQ)
AHCPR Clinical guidelines (on the Web)
AHCPR Conquest
AHCPR Q-SPAN
ANA Nursing Quality Indicators
BASIS-32
Building the Instrument Library. *Medical Outcomes Trust Bulletin.* 5(5) (September):1, 1997.
Child Health Questionnaire (CHQ) (1997). The Child Health Questionnaire: Design and application. *Medical Outcomes Trust Bulletin* 5(3): 1, 4.
European Organization for Research and Treatment of Cancer (EORTC) Study Group on Quality of Life
HEDIS 3.0 Reporting Set Measures
HEDIS 3.0 Testing Set Measures
JCAHO ORYX
London Handicap Scale
Medical Outcomes Trust
MOS-HIV Health Survey (1997). The Medical Outcomes Study–HIV Health Survey (MOS-HIV). *Medical Outcomes Trust Bulletin* 5(1): 2.

NCQA-HEDIS
Pediatric Asthma Quality of Life Questionnaire (PAQLQ)
Quality of Well-Being Scale
Seattle Angina Questionnaire
SF-12 Health Survey
SF-36 Health Survey
Sickness Impact Profile

Additional Bibliography

Bowles, K.H., and M.D. Naylor (1996). Nursing intervention classification systems. *Image: Journal of Nursing Scholarship* 28(4): 303–8.

Boyer, J.G., and J.A.L. Earp (1997). The development of an instrument for assessing the quality of life of people with diabetes: Diabetes-39. *Diabetes* 5(5): 440–53.

Coenen, A., K.D. Marek, and S.P. Lundeen (1996). Using nursing diagnoses to explain utilization in a community nursing center. *Research in Nursing and Health* 19: 441–5.

Delaney, C., and S. Moorhead (1995). The nursing minimum data set, standardized language, and health care quality. *Journal of Nursing Care Quality* 10(1): 16–30.

Essink-Bot, M.L., P.F. Krabbe, G.J. Bonsel, and N.K. Aaronson (1997). An empirical comparison of four generic health status measures: The Nottingham Health Profile, the Medical Outcomes Study 36-Item Short-Form Health Survey, the COOP/WONCA Charts, and the EuroQol Instrument. *Medical Care* 35(5): 522–37.

Heaman, M., and L. Loewen (1997). Outcomes research: an annotated bibliography. *The Manitoba Nursing Research Institute.*

Imbruce, R.P., and J. Selevan (1997). Pharmacoeconomics and the quality of life in the diagnosis and management of asthma: what is your FEEVY? an educational supplement to *The Journal of Care Management.*

Instrument application: quality of well-being scale used to assess treatment intervention. *Medical Outcomes Trust Bulletin* 1: May, 1996.

Kaplan, R.M., C.J. Atkins, and R. Timms (1984). Validity of a quality of well-being scale as an outcome measure in chronic obstructive pulmonary disease. *Journal of Chronic Diseases* 37(2): 85–95.

Kosinski, M. (1997). Scoring the SF-12 Physical and Mental Health Summary measures. *Medical Outcomes Trust Bulletin* 5(5): 3–4.

Maas, M.L., M. Johnson, and S. Moorhead (1996). Classifying nursing-sensitive patient outcomes. *Image: Journal of Nursing Scholarship* 28(4): 295–301.

Marek, K.D. (1996). Nursing diagnoses and home care nursing utilization. *Public Health Nursing* 13(3): 195–200.

Naylor, M.D., B.H. Munro, and D.A. Brooten (1991). Measuring the effectiveness of nursing practice. *Clinical Nurse Specialist* 5(4): 210–15.

Perrin, E.B. (1995) SAC instrument review process. *Medical Outcomes Trust Bulletin* 3(4): September 1.

Prescott, P.A., J.W. Ryan, K.L. Soeken, A.H. Castorr, K.O. Thompson, and C.Y. Phillips (1991). The patient intensity for nursing index: a validity assessment. *Research in Nursing and Health* 14: 213–21.

Schlenker, R.E. (1996). Outcomes across the care continuum: home health care. Center for Health Services Research, University of Colorado Health Sciences Center.

Shaughnessy, P.W., K.S. Crisler, and R.E. Schlenker (1995). Medicare's oasis: standardized outcome and assessment information set for home health care. distributed by the National Association for Home Care.

Sieber, W.J., T. Ganiats, and R. Kaplan (1997). Validation of a self-administered quality of well-being (QWB) scale. *Medical Outcomes Trust Bulletin* 5(5): 2, 4.

Ware, J.E., and C.D. Sherbourne (1992). The MOS 36-item short-form health survey SF-36, I: conceptual framework and item selection. *Medical Care* 30(6): 473–83.

APPENDIX

D

Other Literature Reviewed *(Not Included in Annotated Bibliography)*

Appendix D includes articles that were reviewed but not included in the analysis of indicators because they did not meet the criteria for inclusion.

Anagnos, A., W. McConnell, L. Chafetz, and S. Barto (1993). A consumer-oriented program review process for mental health care. *New Directions for Mental Health Services* 58: 77–84.

Anderson, M.A., K.S. Hanson, N.W. DeVilder, and L.B. Helms (1996). Hospital readmissions during home care: a pilot study. *Journal of Community Health Nursing* 13(1): 1–12.

Badger, T.A., R. Dumas, and T. Kwan (1996). Knowledge of depression and application to practice: a program evaluation. *Issues in Mental Health Nursing* 17(2): 93–109.

Badger, T.A. (1996). Family members' experiences living with members with depression. *Western Journal of Nursing Research* 18(2): 149–71.

Badger, T.A. (1996).Living with depression: family members' experiences and treatment needs. *Journal of Psychosocial Nursing and Mental Health Services* 34(1): 21–29; 48–9.

Baradell, J.G. (1994). Cost-effectiveness and quality of care provided by clinical nurse specialists. *Journal of Psychosocial Nursing* 32(3): 21–4.

Barrell, L.M., E.I. Merwin, and E.C. Poster (1997). Patient outcomes used by advanced practice psychiatric nurses to evaluate effectiveness of practice. *Archives of Psychiatric Nursing* 11(4): 184–97.

Beck, C., B. Baldwin, T. Modlin, and S. Lewis (1990). Caregivers' perception of aggressive behavior in cognitively impaired nursing home residents. *Journal of Neuroscience Nursing* 22(3): 169–72.

Bergstrom, N., B. Braden, M. Kemp, M. Champagne, and E. Ruby (1996). Multi-site study of incidence of pressure ulcers and the relationship between risk level, demographic characteristics, diagnoses, and prescription of preventive interventions. *The American Geriatrics Society Journal* 44: 22–30.

Bergstrom, N., B. Braden, P. Boynton, and S. Bruch (1995). Using a research-based assessment scale in clinical practice. *Nursing Clinics of North America* 30(3): 539–51.

Bolton, L.L., L. Van Rijswijk, and F.A. Shaffer (1996). Quality wound care equals cost-effective wound care. *Nursing Management* 27(7): 30–7.

Braden, B. (1997). Preventing pressure sores. *Home Health Focus* 4(1): 4, 6, 7.

Brooten, D., S. Gennaro, H. Knapp, N. Jovene, L. Brown, and R. York (1991). Functions of the CNS in early discharge and home follow-up of very low birthweight infants. *Clinical Nurse Specialist* 5(4): 196–201.

Brooten, D., S. Kumar, L.P. Brown, P. Butts, S.A. Finkler, S. Bakewell-Sachs, A. Gibbons, and M. Delivoria-Papadopoulos (1986). A randomized clinical trial of early hospital discharge and home follow-up of very low birth-weight infants. *The New England Journal of Medicine* 315(15): 934–9.

Buchner, D.M., M.C. Hornbrook, N.G. Kutner, M.E. Tinetti, M.G. Ory, C.D. Mulrow, K.B. Schechtman, M.B. Gerety, M.A. Fiatarone, S.L. Wolf, J. Rossiter, C. Arfken, K. Kanten, L.A. Lipsitz, R.W. Sattin, L.A. DeNino, and The FICSIT Group (1993). Development of the common data base for the FICSIT trials. *The American Geriatrics Society Journal* 41: 297–308.

Bull, M., L.L., Jervis, and M. Her (1995). Hospitalized elders: the difficulties families encounter. *Journal of Gerontological Nursing* June: 19–23.

Bull, M.J., G. Maruyama, and D. Luo(1995). Testing a model for posthospital transition of family caregivers for elderly persons. *Nursing Research* 44(3): 132–8.

Bull, M.J., and L.J. Jervis (1997). Strategies used by chronically ill older women and their caregiver daughters in managing posthospital care. *Journal of Advanced Nursing* 25: 541–7.

Combes-Orme, T., J. Reis, and L. Dantes Ward (1985). Effectiveness of home visits by public health nurses in maternal and child health: an empirical review. *Public Health Reports* 100(5): 490–9.

Davis, M.A., J.G. Sebastian, and J. Tschetter (1997). Measuring quality of nursing home service: residents' perspective. *Psychological Reports* 81: 531–42.

Doran, K., B. Sampson, R. Staus, C. Ahern, and D. Schiro (1997). Clinical pathway across tertiary and community care after an interventional cardiology procedure. *The Journal of Cardiovascular Nursing* 11(2): 1–14.

Doran-Marek, K. (1998). Measuring the effectiveness of nursing care. *Outcomes Management for Nursing Practice* 1(1): 8–12.

Dunbar, S.B., and J.G. Summerville (1997). Cognitive therapy for ventricular dysrhythmia patients. *The Journal of Cardiovascular Nursing* 12(1): 33–44.

Faucett. J., V. Ellis, P. Underwood, A. Naqvi, and D. Wilson (1990). The effect of Orem's self-care model on nursing care in a nursing home setting. *The Journal of Advanced Nursing* 15: 659–66.

Flaherty, J.H., M. McBride, S. Marzoouk, D.K. Miller, N. Chien, M. Hanchett, S. Leander, F.E. Kaiser, and J.E. Morley (1998). Decreasing hospitalization rates for older home care patients with symptoms of depression. *The American Geriatrics Society Journal* 46(1): 31–8.

Frenn, M., S.P. Lundeen, K.S. Martin, S.K. Riesch, and S.A. Wilson (1996). Symposium on nursing centers: past, present, and future. *Journal of Nursing Education* 35(2): 54–62.

Goodloe, L.R., R.C. Sampson, B. Munjas, T.R. Whitworth, C.D. Lantz, E. Tangley, and W. Miller (1996). Clinical ladder to professional advancement program: an evolutionary process. *Journal of Nursing Administration* 26(6): 58–64.

Graven, S.N., F.W. Bowen, D. Brooten, A. Eaton, M.N. Graven, M. Hack, L.A. Hall, N. Hansen, H. Hurt, R. Kavaljuna, et al (1992). The high risk infant environment, part 2: the role of caregiving and the social environment. *Journal of Perinatology*. XII (3): 267–75.

Harris, D., and E.F., Morrison (1995). Managing violence without coercion. *Archives of Psychiatric Nursing* 9(4): 203–10.

Heacock, P.R., C.M. Beck, E. Souder, and S. Mercer (1997). Assessing dressing ability in dementia. *Geriatric Nursing: American Journal of Care for the Aging* 18(3): 107–11.

Hogan Miller, E., D.A. Nordquist, K.A. Doran, C.K. Ahern, and Y.M. Cariveau Karsten (1998). Interregional healthcare: patient stories and chart reviews. *Clinical Nurse Specialist* 12(1): 15–21.

Howard, P.B., and D. Greiner (1997). Constraints to advanced psychiatric–mental health nursing practice. *Archives of Psychiatric Nursing* XI (4): 198–209.

Johnson, J.E., V.K. Fieler, G.S. Wlasowicz, M.L. Mitchell, and L.S. Jones (1997). The effects of nursing care guided by self-regulation theory on coping with radiation therapy. *Oncology Nursing Forum* 24(6): 1041–50.

Jones, K.R., B.M. Jennings, P. Moritz, and M.T. Moss (1997). Policy issues associated with analyzing outcomes of care. *Image: Journal of Nursing Scholarship* 29(3): 261–7.

Langolis, J.A., G.S. Smith, D.E. Nelson, R.W. Sattin, J.A. Stevens, and C.A. DeVito (1995). Dependence in activities of daily living as a risk factor for fall injury events among older people living in the community. *Journal of the American Geriatric Society* 43: 275–8.

Lundeen, S.P., B. Friedbacher, M. Thomas, and T. Jackson (1997). Testing the viability of collaborative interdisciplinary practice in community-focused primary health care: a case study in change. *Wisconsin Medical Journal* 6(96): 30–6.

MacCovy, S., T. Skinner, and M. Hines (1996). Fall risk assessment tools. *Applied Nursing Research* 9(4): 213–18.

Marek, K.D. (1995) Manual to Develop Guidelines. Washington, DC: American Nurses Publishing.

McCollam, M.E. (1995). Evaluation and implementation of a research-based falls assessment innovation. *Nursing Clinics of North America* 30(3): 507–14.

McDaniel, C. (1990). Reorganization of community psychiatric services by professional nurses. *Issues in Mental Health Nursing* 11: 397–405.

Merwin, E., and A. Mauck (1995). Psychiatric nursing outcome research: the state of the science. *Archives of Psychiatric Nursing* IX(6): 311–31.

Miller, K.E., C.A. King, B.N. Shain, and M.W. Naylor (1992). Suicidal adolescents' perceptions of their family environment. *Suicide and Life-Threatening Behavior* 22(2): 226–39.

Morrison, E.F. (1994). The evolution of a concept: aggression and violence in psychiatric settings. *Archives of Psychiatric Nursing* 8(4): 245–53.

Morrison, E.F. (1993). Toward a better understanding of violence in psychiatric settings: debunking the myths. *Archives of Psychiatric Nursing* 7(6): 328–35.

Murphy, M.F., and M.D. Moller (1993). Relapse management in neurobiological disorders: the Moller-Murphy Symptom Management Assessment Tool. *Archives of Psychiatric Nursing* VII (4): 226–35.

Naylor, M.D., B.H. Munro, and D.A. Brooten (1991). Measuring the effectiveness of nursing practice. *Clinical Nurse Specialist* 5(4): 210–15.

Payne, S.M., D. Campbell, B.G. Penzias, and E. Socholitzky (1992). New methods for evaluating utilization management programs. *Quality Review Bulletin* 18(10): 340–7.

Penticuff, L.M., B. Medhoff-Cooper, D. Brooten, L. Brown (1992). The HOME Scale: the influence of socioeconomic status on the evaluation of the home environment. *Nursing Research* 41(6): 338–41.

Rantz, M. J., G.F. Petroski, R.W. Madsen, J. Scott, D.R. Mehr, L. Popejoy, L.L. Hicks, R. Porter, M. Zwygart-Stauffacher, and V. Grando (1997). Setting thresholds for MDS quality indicators for nursing home quality improvement reports. *Journal on Quality Improvement* 23(11): 602–11.

Sampson, R., and J. Mercier (1998). The professional transitions workshop: cornerstones of practice. *Journal of Nursing Administration* 28(1): 25–9.

Sauer, C.D., and S.M. Ford (1995). Quality, cost-effective psychiatric treatment: a CNS-MD collaborative practice model. *Archives of Psychiatric Nursing* IX(6): 332–7.

Smith, C.E. (1996). Quality of life and caregiving in technological home care. *Annual Review of Nursing Research* 14: 95–118.

Smith, C.E. (1995). Technology and home care. *Annual Review of Nursing Research* 13: 137–67.

Stevens, J.A., K.E. Powell, S.M. Smith, P.A. Wingo, and R.W. Sattin (1997). Physical activity, functional limitations, and the risk of fall-related fractures in the community-dwelling elderly. *Annals of Epidemiology* 7(1): 54–61.

Strumwasser, I., N.V. Paranjpe, D.L. Ronis, D. Share, and L.J. Sell (1990). Reliability and validity of utilization review criteria: appropriateness evaluation protocol, standardized medreview instrument, and intensity-severity-discharge criteria. *Medical Care* 28(2):95–111.

Turkoski, B., L.L. Pierce, S. Schreck, J. Salter, R. Radziewicz, J. Guhde, and R. Bradley (1997). Clinical nursing judgement related to reducing the incidence of falls by elderly patients. *Rehabilitation Nursing* 22(3): 124–30.

White, N. (1996). Illness responses and treatment. *Community Nursing Research* 29: 137–43.

Williams, M.W., and M. Nolan (1993). The prevention of falls among older people at home. *British Journal of Nursing* 2(12): 609–13.

Wiseman, K.C. (1996). Appropriate nursing care for hemodialysis patients with uncomplicated hypotensive events. *ANNA Journal* 32(4): 404–5.

Zachariah, R., and S.P. Lundeen (1997). Research and practice in an academic community nursing center. 29(3): 255–60.

The Journal of Advanced Nursing Practice

Several articles from the above journal were reviewed but did not meet the criteria for inclusion in the analysis of the scientific merit of the indicators. In addition, there are many popular nursing journals that were not in this analysis, because the types of studies that they print did not meet the research criteria that were used. The reviewed literature that was not used was determined unsuitable for this study's purposes for one or more of the following reasons:

1. The research was descriptive in nature.
2. The research was a literature review that did not contain an analysis of the results that were sited or enough detail about the scientific basis of the research to conclude that the analysis of the literature had scientific merit.
3. The sample sizes cited in the studies published were not large enough to generate conclusive results.

Some of the articles that were reviewed in these journals were used to identify other literature that was reviewed or to provide a theoretical basis for inclusion of indicators in the analysis.

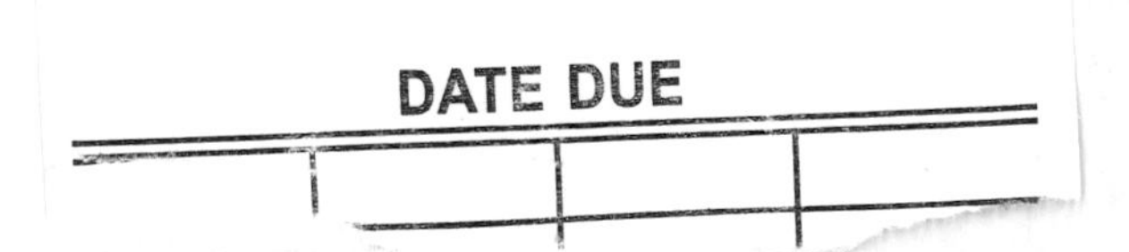
DATE DUE